Straight Talk Scoliosis – The Journey Continues

Testimonials

"*Straight Talk Scoliosis, The Journey Continues* offers a wealth of information and support to anyone dealing with scoliosis. As someone who wore a brace throughout my childhood, I wish I'd had access to a book like this when I was growing up. I'm thrilled this book exists now to help children and their families navigate their treatment and, importantly, to know that they're not alone."

— Rachel Rabkin Peachman
Health Journalist

"It is my wish that newly diagnosed families will read this edition of *Straight Talk Scoliosis* before venturing on their journey. Consistent with our philosophy of looking at the person and not just the curve, *The Journey Continues* speaks to the perspective of 'patient as person.' Terry and Robin are comprehensive in their efforts to help each child and parent be both informed and seen as a whole person. This book is written from the hearts and minds of people who have been there and want to make your journey go a bit smoother."

— Manuel Rigo, MD, PhD
Chair of Barcelona Scoliosis Physical Therapy School

Your child was just diagnosed with scoliosis ... *Now what?*
"*Straight Talk Scoliosis, The Journey Continues* takes you beyond the Cobb angle as it addresses the 'other side' of the scoliosis journey – the confusion, challenges, and alternative treatments.

As moms of daughters with scoliosis, they bring this information to you from personal experience, along with their ongoing relationship with the scoliosis medical community over the past 15 years. Terry and Robin are real people, with real-life experience, who understand the diagnosis and the journey ahead. This book reads as if you are sitting down and talking with the individuals themselves, while raising awareness as to the questions you need to be asking.

Eight years ago, my daughter Abbey was diagnosed with AIS. I was fortunate to find Curvy Girls and the first edition of this book, *Straight Talk With The Curvy Girls*, within a few months of her diagnosis. I know that the Curvy Girls organization and the *Straight Talk* book has changed my daughter's scoliosis journey, and my 'Mom journey' for the better.

Thank you Robin, Leah, Terry and Rachel for your continued dedication and commitment to helping girls and their families navigate this scoliosis journey. You have touched SO MANY lives; my daughter being one of them."

— Sebrina Cronin
Parent

Straight Talk Scoliosis – The Journey Continues

Theresa E. Mulvaney
Robin Stoltz, LCSW

Straight Talk Scoliosis the Journey Continues

Copyright © 2021, Theresa E. Mulvaney and Robin Stoltz, LCSW

All rights reserved. No part of this book may be reproduced, stored in a retrieval system, or transmitted in any form or by any means electronic, mechanical, photocopying, recording, or otherwise, without the written permission of the publisher.

Published by: Straight Talk Scoliosis, LLC
Designed by Tom Emmerson, Alternative Graphic Solutions, Inc.
Illustrations: Jenna Stern and Glenda Andrea Torasso

ISBN: 978-0-9888231-1-2

Medical Disclaimer: The information contained herein reflects only the opinions of the authors and is not intended as medical advice or a substitution for medical counseling. The current book is designed for educational purposes only and is not engaged in rendering medical advice or professional services. It is not intended nor implied to be a substitute for professional medical advice. The information provided herein should not be used for diagnosing or treating a health problem or a disease. It is not a substitute for professional care. Anyone using this book is advised to consult with a physician regarding personal medical care. If you have or suspect you may have a health problem, consult your healthcare provider. Reading this book does not create a physician-patient relationship.

Information contained in this book is for informational purposes only, and readers and viewers should consult a medical professional before beginning any course of action based on the topics covered in the source. Some of the activities described may be too strenuous or not appropriate for some people and the reader(s) should consult a physician before engaging in them.

Disclaimer: We have made every effort to insure that content is accurate, correct and current, and we are not liable for any unintentional errors. Mention of specific companies, organizations, authorities or medical professionals does not imply endorsement of them and we are not responsible or liable for their information and contents, nor does it imply their endorsement of this Book.
Under no circumstances, shall the authors and publishers be liable under any theory of recovery for any damages arising out of or in any manner connected with the use of information, services, or documents from the site.
Where we have received permission we have used real names but some names and identifying details, as well as identifying characteristics and details such as physical properties, occupations and places of residence have been changed to protect the privacy of individuals.

Printed in the United States of America
This book is printed on acid-free paper

*For his endless dedication and lifelong work
advocating for patients in the world of scoliosis,
we'd like to dedicate this book to*
Joe O'Brien
President, CEO of National Scoliosis Foundation

To Leah and Rachel who brought us on this journey

Contents

And The Journey Continues...   xvii
Prologue: Secrets   xx

Part 1: Memoirs   1

Leah Stoltz and her mother, Robin Stoltz
Coming Full Circle —Leah   3
Adolescence or Scoliosis? —Robin   22

Rachel Mulvaney and her mother, Terry Mulvaney
I Wouldn't Change a Thing —Rachel and Terry   31

Mimi Macklin and her mother, Julie Macklin
Finding the Magic —Mimi and Julie   51

Alyssa Dunlop and her mother, Jusna Dunlop
My Kind of Normal —Alyssa   63
Hope House —Jusna   72

Jamiah Bennett and her mother, Cynthia Parker
The Power Within —Jamiah and Cynthia   82

Katelyn Winkler and her mother, Amy Winkler
Twisted Road —Katelyn   92
It Started with a Book —Amy   99

Intisar Mughal and her mother, Shahida Mohamed
Mama Has Your Back —Intisar and Shahida   106

Sophie Klein and her mother, Cara Harth
The Strength Within —Sophie   119
Guilt, Anxiety and Resilience —Cara   128

Part 2: Taking Charge: TeenTalk   135
A Message from Leah   136
A Message from Rachel   137

EmBracing Fashion – Rachel's Tips	138
A Brace ... Are They Crazy?	143
School Nurse Letter	148
Bone Nutrition Trivia	150
Leah's Surgery Tips	151
Taking "Back" Control	156

Part 3: Parent Support — 173

Signs and Symptoms of Scoliosis	174
Five Stages of Coping with Scoliosis	175
Preparing for Your Child's Medical Visit	180
What if Your Child Needs Surgery?	184
Advocating for Your Child in The School System	192

Part 4: Understanding the World of Bracing — 197

Mike Mangino, CPO, CPed	198
Bay Orthopedics and Rehabilitation, NY	
Luke Strikleather, CPO	203
National Scoliosis Center, VA	
Grant Wood, MS, CPO, CO	210
Align Clinic, CA	
Jim Wynne, CPO, FAAOP	215
Boston Orthotics & Prosthetics, MA	

Part 5: Physiotherapy Scoliosis Specific Exercises — 221

Rigo Method	
Beth Janssen, PT, WI	222
Setting It Straight	
Marissa Muccio, PT, SC	234
Introduction to SEAS	
Stefano Negrini, MD, Milan, Italy	239

Part 6: Straight Talk — 247

Discussions with Orthopedists — 248
James Barci, MD — 248
  Stony Brook University Children's Hospital, NY
A. Noelle Larson, MD — 254
  Mayo Clinic, MN
Michael Vitale, MD, MPH — 260
  Pediatric Orthopaedics, NYP Hospital, NY
Laurence E. Mermelstein, MD — 265
  Long Island Spine Specialists, NY
Nigel Price, MD, FAAOS, FAAP — 272
  Children's Mercy, MO
Craig Eberson, MD — 275
  University Orthopedics, RI

Fusionless Surgeries — 278
Vertebral Body Tethering
  Joshua Pahys, MD — 278
    Shriners Hospitals for Children, PA
ApiFix
  Nigel Price, MD — 284
    Children's Mercy Hospital, MO

Connecting the Dots — 288
Understanding Postural Orthostatic Tachycardia Syndrome (POTS) and Ehlers-Danlos Syndrome (EDS)
  Phil Fischer, MD — 288
    Mayo Clinic, MN

Low-Dose Radiation — 292
EOS imaging system
  Dana Goldy, RT — 292

Part 7: Psychological Support and Guidance   **297**
   Robin Stoltz, LCSW
     Behavioral Health, NY
   Learning from Adversity: Twist of Fate   298
   Communication 101   301
   Seeking Support   303
   Choosing a Mental Health Professional   304

Final Thoughts   **305**
   Our Work Is Not Done   306
   Scoliosis Glossary   308
   Acknowledgements   311
   Meet the Authors   314

Foreword

This is an honor for me to be asked to write this foreword about Robin and Terry's precious book, **Straight Talk Scoliosis – The Journey Continues.** I am not an orthopedic surgeon, nor researcher, but a simple clinician that has been working for the past 35 years exclusively in the field of scoliosis rehabilitation— bracing and Physiotherapy Scoliosis Specific Exercises (PSSE). During these years, the practice of medicine has changed quite a bit. There are two emerging models with increased popularity in the healthcare community—Informed Evidence Based Medicine Model (EBM) and the Biopsychosocial Model, two concepts which are made evident throughout this book.

Through well-designed interviews with renowned specialists, this book provides valuable information regarding several treatment options in accordance with the Informed Evidence Based Model. In addition, the support of personal stories and messages enlightens the importance of the 'biopsychosocial model.' The message from Rachel, summarizes in a simple, concise and perfect way what is behind this model: *"The numeric value of your curve degree does NOT define you. Remember, an X-ray will only generate a number; however, it is up to you to determine how that number will impact you. Do not allow a number to make you feel less than."* Rachel's message speaks perfectly to this idea that I try to emphasize throughout the Barcelona Scoliosis Physiotherapist School (BSPTS), "Looking after the person, not just the curve."

Scoliosis is a lifelong condition in that once developed, you will need to learn coping skills. There is no "magic solution" that can change you into a person without scoliosis, but what we can offer is viable therapy options to diminish the impact of the scoliosis on your physical and mental health. Whether you are an operated or non-operated patient, you need to learn how to cope and accept the condition. That is one of the many topics that *Straight Talk Scoliosis – The Journey Continues,* approaches very well.

Like my dear colleague and friend Dr. Stefano Negrini says in his interview, *"This is the field that manages the disability and rehabilitation of spinal disorders. This is the field of deep complexity."* Scoliosis is a condition that encompasses multiple clinical presentations in relation to: age of onset, causation, curvature pattern, risk of progression, response to treatment, and impact on quality of life for today, tomorrow and into the future. However, quality of life is not necessarily determined by scoliosis itself, nor is it restricted to a simple radiograph or an angular value.

Please, allow me to tell you a short story, with an imaginary protagonist who represents so many of the young girls I have seen through the years. It is an old story that continues to resonate in contemporary times:

Isabel is sitting in front of me, beside her is mom and dad. They came into my office room about 35 minutes ago. They told me about Isabel's scoliosis being detected when she was 11. She is now 16 and has a major scoliosis curve. She is fully mature. She did not receive any specific treatment or care. She was followed until she was 13, starting under 20° and then reaching 32°– still at Risser 0, already post-menarche. She had been threatened with a brace several times—this is the correct word, "threatened" but even after reaching 32° her doctor was against bracing. NO explanations about her condition, what a brace is, or potential risks. Isabel's parents were not informed about the implications of maturation in relation to scoliosis; they were just told "no more risk once she is mature." So, they interpreted Isabel as mature after starting her menses, and asked themselves, "Why continue doing radiographs every six months for nothing?" and, consequently, stopped bringing Isabel for X-rays. Three years later, her parents observed she was noticeably imbalanced and her waist-pelvis asymmetry had significantly worsened. Once again, they sought out care.

After so many years, still now, more than ever, I feel a lump in my throat when I look at the eyes of a girl like Isabel and have to explain to her what has happened. This is a clear example of "undertreatment" but how to approach this situation without hurting Isabel more? We will need to have a long conversation. Too many things to explain about why we are left with the options that she is now facing today—an operation or accepting the condition as is. She could do specific physiotherapy for life as a palliative treatment, or simply accept her scoliosis and do nothing. Unfortunately, now there are limited options. Which will be the best option for Isabel? Honesty, who knows for sure.

One thing is clear, we cannot prevent progression every time we treat using a brace and PSSE. But it also does not help if you have not been given all the information or given a personal opinion of a doctor who says, "I do not believe in bracing" or "I do not think a brace will prevent anything." Follow the research and evidence! There is clear evidence that bracing works. Although certainly, we still need to learn about improving our braces, being better in selecting the patient we treat with a brace, and improving the response to the brace.

It is absolutely normal that patients would like to hear that an operation is not necessary. In some cases, delaying surgery can be the wrong decision as this too falls into the category of undertreatment. The border between undertreatment and overtreatment in this field is a thin line. The final decision belongs to the patient and family.

As part of the general information provided by this book, you will find specific names related to the PSSE techniques, brace types, and surgical interventions. The EBM Model relies on the balance of all three components: external evidence, clinical experience and patient preferences, in order to make a most informed decision. In *The Journey Continues* you will be reminded of the importance of being part of a team. Do your due diligence through research and preparation, and by sharing all the necessary information to facilitate a consensus about your best possible treatment options. It is important to collect information before jumping into any specific type of treatment.

Presently, there is evidence that PSSE helps the brace work more effectively, aside from other well-known benefits. These benefits need to be well explained to prevent false expectations. It needs to be clarified that no brace or PSSE technique produces an automatic result just for the given name, such as Rigo Cheneau, Schroth, Boston Brace, SEAS, etc. It is the knowledge, experience and personal skills of the provider that is more important than the name itself.

Finally, remember also the words from Rachel, *'Throughout my scoliosis journey, I allowed the results of my X-ray to dictate my self-esteem and determine how I measured "success." If my curves worsened, I thought I "failed" bracing or my Schroth Method exercises. During these years I put an enormous amount of pressure on myself, which was both unrealistic and unfair."*

Maybe, the story about this imaginary girl called Isabel, would have been completely different if she, or her parents (or her doctor?) would have had the chance of reading this present edition of **Straight Talk Scoliosis – *The Journey Continues*.**

— Manuel Rigo, MD, PhD
Medical Director of the Institute Rigo Quera Salva S.L.P.
Chair of the Barcelona Scoliosis Physical Therapy School - BSPTS

And the Journey Continues...

When our daughters were first diagnosed, we thought scoliosis was something they would grow out of, not grow up with. Having the realization that scoliosis is a lifelong condition began our personal mission for better solutions and ultimately the writing of *Straight Talk with the Curvy Girls* first edition, and *Straight Talk Scoliosis – The Journey Continues*.

There are many unknowns and variables associated with scoliosis that can easily overwhelm parents and children—rate of curve progression, length and types of treatment, aggressive versus conservative approaches, and worse, false claims about quick cures and miracle solutions that prey on our vulnerability and our wallets. The reality is that there is no quick fix, bracing *is* effective and should not be abandoned for the promise of something more or less or different. To date there is no cure for scoliosis and if it's a quick fix, buyer beware. We caution you to not waste precious time and money on unproven methods. Follow the standard of care.

It is our aim to provide readers with reputable treatments, encouragement, and the skills necessary to deal with the special challenges for scoliosis-involved families. Our work has been informed from countless meetings of Curvy Girls' chapters, medical conferences, as well as conventions held by the organization. We have listened to the questions being asked by girls with scoliosis and their parents—and taken it all to heart as we worked on this book. We sought out some of the best experts in their fields to answer questions from people just like you. Our goal is singular: To provide families with the best information available.

Once empowered with information, parents' frustrations and sense of powerlessness seem to dissipate. Robin's professional insight into the psychological issues of pre-adolescents, together with Terry's determined call to find answers in mainstream and complementary science beyond the common "wait-and-see" approach, provide those insights and solutions.

CURVY GIRLS SUPPORT

The impact of scoliosis is so much more than what is seen on an X-ray. As a three-dimensional spine condition treated with an orthosis, scoliosis-specific exercises, and/or surgery, the psychosocial impact of scoliosis on teens is often overlooked. Borne of thirteen-year-old Leah Stoltz's hope to connect with other girls experiencing the concerns associated with Adolescent Idiopathic Scoliosis (AIS), Curvy Girls support groups have been effectively serving these needs since 2006.

Leah and her group members reclaim what their scoliosis was threatening to take away—their sense of self-control and overall self-image. Girls who came in thinking that they were alone in their struggle with scoliosis connected with other girls facing similar challenges. The desire to speak with others dealing with the impact of this condition speaks to every child's need to have their scoliosis addressed from a psychological and social standpoint.

Since first assembling, Curvy Girls has welcomed hundreds of girls and their families who, like us, were looking everywhere for guidance and support. It has been our experience that scoliosis-involved families are hungry for information. After diagnosis, they soon find themselves drowning in the hypothetical: *Why wasn't I told that?* or *If I only knew.* In rooms separate from the Girls' meetings, parents commonly, and tearfully, share their guilt or regret for not having intervened sooner, for not pursuing the right information, or for refraining from advocating in some way on their child's behalf. These are just a few of the sentiments that are echoed over and over that became the catalyst for writing our books.

HOW TO READ THIS BOOK

As Straight Talk's journey continues, it is our aim to provide readers with the latest information and advancements in the treatment of scoliosis. We know there is a good deal of information contained in these pages. The memoirs are inspirational in nature and intended to help give teens and their parents the strength and fortitude to continue. You'll see that girls and their parents overcame the challenges they encountered and emerged stronger, more passionate and more vocal in the end.

You needn't begin your Straight Talk journey on page one but instead look at the contents page to choose topics of interest and relevance to you. If bracing, your child will want to read the stories from Rachel, Alyssa, Katelyn, and Sophie. Those anticipating surgery will want to read the memoirs from Leah, Mimi, Jamiah, and Intisar, as well as the section on Preparing for Surgery. Grab a highlighter and take notes. Take a few days to process what you've learned and then share with your child. Knowledge is power and our ultimate goal is for you to be empowered.

NEW DEVELOPMENTS

For returning readers, in addition to new memoirs, the medical section has been expanded in both breadth and depth to include more medical perspectives, as well as new technologies and treatments. Since learning about the Schroth Method while writing the first edition, Curvy Girls championed by Terry and Rachel Mulvaney have worked tirelessly advocating for Scoliosis Specific Exercises to take its rightful place as a conservative care tool in the US. While we've seen some success with Schroth, Rigo Method and the Seas Approach becoming household words among patients, families and medical professionals, we believe there is more to be done. Insurance companies, long mired in the past, need to update their protocols and recognize that these conservative care options are a viable treatment for scoliosis and should be fully covered by insurance—just like the cost of a new brace or spinal surgery. In addition, we have made a concerted effort to educate and inform parents about the existence of low-dose X-ray technology and advocate for its availability to all families.

As we continue our journey, we hope to enable future generations of families affected with scoliosis to have a new, clear protocol for the standard of care. After all, don't we owe it to our children to pursue the safest, most effective treatment!

Prologue: Secrets

They eat away and gnaw at you. Secrets aren't healthy. Secrets develop when you think you have something to hide, something that causes you to feel embarrassment or shame. Because teens may feel embarrassed by having scoliosis or having to wear a brace, they tend to keep both a secret.

Everything begins to change during the teen years—bodies, relationships, and a sense of self. Cognitive capacities expand, hormones begin to affect previously rational thinking selves, and parents may no longer be experienced as a safe haven, maybe even crossing over into enemy territory. All of this is normal in the context of emerging adolescence, although it feels anything but while in the midst of this upheaval.

The major developmental task of adolescence is individuation— establishing one's own identity on the road to independence—which requires teens to pull away from parents and begin to align with peers. Enter scoliosis. Bracing complicates this process, as an adolescent's sense of self can literally become distorted from wearing a brace. The brace challenges self-esteem and can leave teens in a developmental limbo, no longer fully dependent upon parents, yet in fear of rejection from peers.

Middle schoolers go to great lengths to fit in. If fitting in means denying scoliosis, then they may do just that, by refusing to talk about it or even refuse to wear the brace. Because the effects of scoliosis are not necessarily obvious to the naked eye, keeping scoliosis a secret may seem easy at first. Add a body brace into the mix, and the *secret* becomes more difficult to maintain.

"I'm ashamed of wearing a brace. I'm embarrassed to wear this clunky plastic armor around my body. If it were normal, then everyone would wear one. I'm different. Better not let anyone know so they don't think I'm weird." The reality is that others will only think it's weird if you do. Seven new Curvy Girls came to a group meeting and no one could tell the difference between the girls wearing a brace and those that weren't. When we believe something is strange, we tend to act as if it is and then our embarrassment may give away our secret. Now there are two secrets: Scoliosis encased in a brace, and shame.

Each child deals differently with the challenges of wearing a brace. We've seen a few common scenarios: teens who wear their brace and are comfortable sharing with friends, those that outright refuse to wear their brace, those that pretend to wear it and remove it while at school, and others who dutifully wear their brace and hope no one notices. The latter is not a realistic expectation because while most braces are often well hidden under clothing, the act of lifting an arm, bending, or getting clothing caught in a chair holds the potential for exposing the *secret*. The effort it takes to maintain a secret is emotionally exhausting.

So girls, if you're embarrassed over having to wear a brace, you need to come up with some good responses to, "What is that?" One very sophisticated eleven-year-old offers this as an explanation, "I got into a skydiving accident." What does that convey? That statement says, "I am not ashamed." Because she uses humor, she demonstrates a sense of confidence. Maybe that also says not to mess with her. But this may not be your style. Just as Leah tells the Curvy Girls, you have to find your own voice. Think about what will work best for you when someone accidentally knocks into your *abs of steel*.

Practice your response with a trusted friend or family member. Leah's older brother, Paul, teased her all the time about her brace. It gave her good practice! Initially, I got mad that he was making her feel badly about herself and tried to intervene. That didn't stop him. Years later, he told us that he was just trying to bring a little levity into the situation, hoping it would help her deal with kids' comments. I guess he was worried too.

Consider sharing your secret with trusted friends or maybe naming your brace as Rachel did. Some parents have organized brace reveal parties, whereby bracing is introduced in a fun and accepting atmosphere. Since pretending that your brace doesn't exist wears at your self-esteem, it's important to find a way to talk about it.

When you put so much mental energy into thinking about how to keep your brace from being seen or inadvertently touched — like hugging or being bumped into at school — it weighs heavy on your mind. Feeling different can be channeled into a positive direction once you speak openly about your scoliosis. Curvy Girls works on helping kids to understand that scoliosis is nothing to be ashamed of, and that if they share their *secret* they will lighten their load.

> Secrets are burdensome,
> and shame is damaging
> to one's spirit.

The psychological impact of scoliosis and bracing on a teen is much different than on younger children. When a young child wears a brace, she may even feel proud.

One six-year-old came to her first group meeting all smiles. She couldn't wait to show us her tattooed brace. We had just finished making our introductions when she proudly pulled up her shirt to reveal multi-colored butterflies adorning her Boston brace. We oohed and aahed. She wanted to wear the brace on the outside of her shirt so everyone could see. After all, why would one want to hide those beautiful butterflies? Then there is seven-year-old Dana who joined fifteen teens and preteens for her first Curvy Girls group meeting. She listened intently to the girls as they recounted the trials and tribulations of wearing a brace, until she could take no more and announced, "I like my brace. My brace is going to help me and I want to wear it." We all need to take a lesson from the spirit of a child, yet as parents, we have all watched as our child's spirit fades into an adolescent cocoon where we are on the outside looking in.

Adolescence: The time between being a dependent child and an independent adult. Here is where lessons for adulthood are learned.

Her brace
Went on
Her heart
It sank

Inside
Her
Plastic
Shell

Silently
She
Recoiled
In
Self
Despair

Her
World
Consumed
With
Worry
Overcome
With useless
Shame

A voice
Quieted
By a
Secret
Blame

A Spirit
Lost
And
Then
Reclaimed

She shouts
You will
Not
Silence
Me!

More Together Than Alone

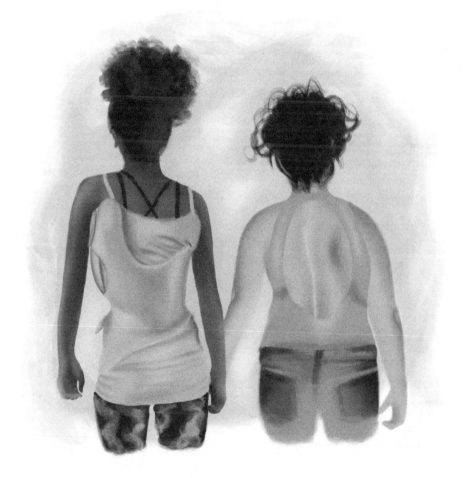

Meet the Curvy Girls

PART 1

Memoirs

As no two curve patterns are alike, neither are the stories carried on the backs of the girls who are telling them. Each girl's story is unique, and the path that each family found in dealing with scoliosis, is different. But in all these different stories we hear strength, courage, and determination. We hope these stories will help empower you during your own scoliosis journey. We hope you, too, will learn that strength can be found, regardless of the curves that life may throw at you. These memoirs inspired us, and we hope that they will be a source of inspiration for you, as well.

Curvy Girls are triumphant all over the world, and you can be too!

Leah

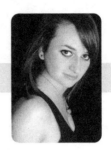

Meet Leah from Long Island

Age: 17

Braced at age 11

Spinal fusion surgery—age 14

Leah started the first teen-run scoliosis support group in 2006 because she wanted to talk with other kids who were going through the same thing.

Leah loves to dance and play golf. She also enjoys reading and traveling.

Curvy Girls has been a way for her to feel supported and give support back to others; it's never having to feel alone.

Leah's story speaks to her resilience. How does a kid make sense of doing all the "right" things, only to end up having to face their ultimate fear? What could have been a tale of victimization, depression, and a teen's sense that it was the end of her world, became a story of triumph... and, ultimately, a gift for others.

Leah's Message: Remember, it's not how big of a challenge you are given that matters, it's how you overcome it. Don't let scoliosis define or defeat you!

Part 1: Memoirs

Leah Stoltz and her mother, Robin Stoltz

Coming Full Circle

Leah

Everything was spinning. Two thousand kids were shouting but I couldn't hear them. A tiara was placed on my head and a bouquet of red roses in my hands. "Breathe, Leah, breathe!" said Nick Cannon, the Chairman of the TeenNick Television Network, as he wrapped his arm around my shoulders and put a microphone in front of my face. I probably wouldn't believe this memory was real if there hadn't been a film crew to record every moment.

"I'm here to give back to someone who's been giving back her entire life," Cannon announced.

Tears started streaming down my face; I couldn't believe he was talking about me!

The year was 2009 and I was standing on the stage with Nick Cannon for the annual TeenNick HALO, or Helping and Leading Others, Award. It was one of the most amazing, and memorable, moments of my life, and it changed my life forever. It all started with my scoliosis diagnosis.

I vaguely recall being told I had scoliosis, a disease that left me with two titanium rods and 22 screws in my back. However, it was that fateful doctor's visit when I was eleven and a half years old that changed my life. I was finishing my first year of middle school when the curve in my spine began to consume my world. I wasn't happy. My body had betrayed me; I didn't feel normal. But who would be happy having to wear a back brace for twenty-two hours a day, seven days a week, for two and a half years?

MY DIAGNOSIS

I believe that I diagnosed myself. None of the school nurses or my pediatrician had noticed, but one day I was scratching around the middle of my back and something felt strange. My spine was twisted under my fingers. I asked my mom to look at it, which she did. A few days later we went for my annual check-up. During my physical exam, I showed my doctor what I had found. He said that if it was anything, it was a very minor scoliosis curve of possibly 5°. That wasn't a good enough answer for my mom. She pointed out the distinctive "S" my spinal column formed. He took out a scoliometer and ran it down the middle of my back. Again, he said it didn't really look like much, but if we wanted, he would give us a referral to an orthopedist.

The following week when we went to see the orthopedist, Dr. Laurence Mermelstein, he said, "Definitely not 5°, probably closer to about 15°." But when I was X-rayed, the result was far from either estimate.

"This is why we take X-rays," Dr. Mermelstein explained. "Sometimes scoliosis just doesn't show."

I had two curves. My main curve in my lower back was 37° with a secondary or compensatory curve of 26° in my upper back. I was immediately thrown into a brace on June 11th, my mom's 49th birthday.

Sixth grade was probably the worst year for me. My best friend of roughly ten years dropped me cold and, at the end of that school year, I was diagnosed with scoliosis. Facing scoliosis without a best friend to talk to left me feeling extremely lonely. Then I was thrown into IT—my brace. IT was that plastic thing staring at me from my orthotist Mike Mangino's hands. How was it possible for anyone to wear IT? I felt like the world wanted to keep me down. There were two weeks left in sixth grade and I couldn't imagine how I would show up to school with IT around my body. Dr. Mike, as I liked to call him, told me that I would ease into it, so I didn't have to wear it all day until I got used to how it felt. I wore IT when I came home from school and on the weekends. Once school was over, I wore it all day to summer camp. And boy was it hot that summer! I kept it a secret. Only one other person besides my camp counselor and nurse knew about it, and that was only so she could help me take it on and off before and after swimming. I loved swimming that summer because it was my only real time out of the brace and I felt...well...normal.

FINDING THE RIGHT CLOTHES

The weekend after I got my brace was *the* horrid shopping trip. Trying to find clothes that would fit over the dreaded brace was an exercise in futility. I remember quite vividly being in the dressing room of Aeropostale® with my aunt, who made a special trip from Florida to take me on this shopping spree. Around me in the dressing room were clothes two sizes too big. I just could not take it any longer. I had tried on outfit after outfit and did not want to look in the mirror one more time to see how awkward I still looked.

I cried, "They don't fit. They don't look right. I can't do this! You can still see the brace. I look like a freak!" I felt completely hopeless.

This was no longer my body but a body the brace formed. I continued crying as I looked at my reflection, disgusted. I soon learned that the flimsy materials that trendy clothes were made from quickly tore as a result of rubbing against the brace. Some of my new clothes were getting ruined. I needed to learn how to check the material for stiffness and thickness in order for it to endure the wear and tear of my brace.

> Having to wear a plastic encasement for hours on end, with no end in sight, felt like the end of the world to me as a twelve-year-old.

Then there was changing for gym class and fearing exposure. One of the challenges of wearing a brace to school was how I would get it off and on without anybody noticing. I could leave early from the class before, but I didn't want to call attention to myself. I ended up shamefully changing in the nurse's office supply closet or bathroom, and consequently arriving late for gym class. After gym, I did my best to change quickly back into my brace and clothes. Although the nurse never had a problem with giving me a late pass, I didn't want to call more attention to myself by walking into class late. In order to do all this, I had to get special consideration in school, which required a meeting and an IEP (individualized education plan), all of which made me feel different. I wanted to hide my brace and keep my scoliosis a secret from my secluded middle school world.

Wearing a brace changed the way I used my body. I could not bend down or move side to side. If I dropped something, I had to leave it on the floor hoping someone would pick it up for me. I was always outgoing, but out of self-consciousness I started to keep to myself.

After building up to full-time bracing, I wore my brace faithfully every day for twenty-two hours. My parents didn't even have to remind me. Two months into bracing, my parents surprised me when they said that my dad was going to take me to get a puppy. Being as responsible as I was with wearing and taking care of my brace showed them that I would be just as responsible taking care of the dog I always wanted.

MY SPINECOR® EXPERIENCE

A few weeks after wearing the Boston Brace, my school nurse told us she had just learned about a girl who, while braced in a soft brace called SpineCor,® had a decrease in her curve. Since a decrease in a curve when out of the brace was unheard of, my mother wanted to find out more. This was the first of numerous orthopedic consults we attended in the following years.

I was greeted with my choice of lollipops, and after looking at the X-rays we brought with us, the orthopedist told us several things. One, my curve was smaller than the 37° we were told; two, I was still not a candidate for the SpineCor® brace because it's not recommended for curves that exceed 24°; and three, there was no reason to be wearing my brace for twenty-two hours; I should only wear it for sixteen hours a day. She said that research shows that bracing at sixteen hours was just as effective as twenty-two hours. So let's see, my curve was smaller, brace time less, and I could have a lollipop of my choosing. Now this was a doctor!

Although it was not recommended, we did go for a consult with an orthotist who carried the SpineCor® brace. I took one look at all those straps and said, "No way am I wearing that!" I could never maneuver the straps in order to go to the bathroom. We returned to Dr. Mermelstein to discuss "Lollipop Doc's" recommendations. Dr. Mermelstein stood by his original recommendation of twenty-two hours, saying that while statistics from a study showed that twenty-two hours of brace wear was no more effective than sixteen hours, this was merely an average of many brace wearers. Some kids fared better with sixteen hours and others with more. But who wanted to take the chance that I would be the one who needed the twenty-two hours. It was too risky, so I continued with the twenty-two-hour regime.

NEW YORK CITY

A year and a half after bracing began, my primary curve had gone from 37° to 47°. Because it was a slow increase over a year's time, my orthopedist was not alarmed. If my curves remained relatively stable and my body didn't grow more, he felt satisfied that I would not need surgery. However, someone suggested to my mom that we should go to a particular orthopedist in Manhattan for his opinion. Since this was at a renowned children's hospital, his opinion would of course be one of the best. It's a curious thing about "the best." We learned that what might be the best for one person is not necessarily what is best suited for another.

My mom and I drove into Manhattan during the holiday season when the City is quite beautiful but very cold. She promised we would go to the ballet, Swan Lake, when we were done with our appointment. My parents always did something to make a consultation special.

The orthopedist at the hospital interviewed us before sending us downstairs for X-rays. We came with our own digital X-rays on a computerized disc but he said they like to take their own. So we waited downstairs in the bowels of the hospital for the "special" X-rays to be taken. Then we waited an hour for them to be developed before returning upstairs with them. He looked at my full-length X-rays, which were divided into three separate films and said we could consider not wearing the brace any longer. Boy, are these special X-rays! He went on to explain that research shows that bracing curves in the 40° range is less effective. Now don't get excited and throw away your braces after reading this because this too is "just a statistic." Many kids wear braces for curves that are more than 40° and can have a good result.

The next question my mom asked was that if we choose to continue with bracing, which we both agreed I should do, did he think my current brace was sufficient? He then took us across the hall and left us with the orthotist, who took one look at my brace and deemed it completely ineffective. Wearing only my underwear and a bra with a tank top they gave me; he proceeded to push and pull me into wet gauze. My mom was sitting there filling out papers and I'm standing in the middle of this very large room while a guy who I could barely understand was covering my torso in gauze to fit me for a brand new brace. To make matters worse, he was sitting in a chair with wheels and kept running over my toes. My winces were met with more pulling and pushing. Then the worst thing happened. This guy began to wrap my chest in the wet gauze. I had no idea what was going on, and neither did my mom until I tearfully called out to her. We exchanged a very confused glance. My mother insisted he stop what he was doing and bring in the doctor. We didn't even understand why they were fitting me for a new brace that was more restrictive then the first, when the doctor said I didn't even need one anymore. I refused to wear any brace that covered my chest. He reluctantly agreed to make it under my breastbone, all the while going on about how this was not the right way to do it.

From that day on, we have never gone to a doctor's appointment without asking tons of questions first. We never wanted to be in a situation that wasn't planned for. My mom and I also learned later on that the brace company was not part of the hospital but a separate company with offices closer to where I lived. So when the new brace was completed, the owner of the company brought the brace to my house.

After wearing this new brace for a couple of days, the owner met me at my follow-up visit with my own orthopedist, Dr. Mermelstein, who told him what needed to be adjusted. When I returned to Dr. Mermelstein with the fixed brace, he noted that it was made incorrectly; it was the exact opposite of what it should have been. This meant it was pushing where it shouldn't and not pushing where it should. Dr. Mermelstein called our original orthotist Dr. Mike, and asked that we be seen right away for a new brace fitting. Dr. Mike made up a new brace and I wore that one until I no longer wore a brace.

BREAKING THE SECRET

This secret showed no matter how hard I tried to keep it hidden. The thing about adolescent idiopathic scoliosis (AIS) is that it usually happens during middle school—a time when you worry most about fitting in. I felt embarrassed about having to wear a brace to school.

Between worrying about being bumped into in the hallway, not being able to bend down, and having to change for gym class, my scoliosis was a burden. AIS is our big secret. I wanted to hide it from my world, and with the exception of my school nurse and gym teacher that was exactly what I planned to do. I told no one outside of my family—until an eighth-grade biology presentation when the timing felt right to me.

Topics were randomly picked out of a bowl. Ms. Fitzpatrick told us there was no swapping; whatever topic we picked was ours to keep. I picked "pneumonia." Then, I waited until the end of class and approached my teacher. I raised my shirt slightly so she could peek at my plastic torso and asked if I could report on scoliosis. Her encouragement was the turning point in my secret brace life.

On the day of the presentation, I walked into class carrying my brace in my hands and I used an overhead projector to project my X-rays on the wall in a larger-than-life image. All eyes were on me as I explained what scoliosis looked like inside and out. It wasn't until I learned how to share my "secret" that I could return to my outgoing self. Now, if someone asked why I couldn't bend to pick up their pencil, I could tell them. If a kid knocked into me in the hallway, I could respond with, "Abs of steel. Feel 'em."

STARTING CURVY GIRLS

Although it is a common disorder, I found myself without anyone to whom I could relate. I was in the eighth grade when we located a scoliosis support group held at a local hospital. My mother insisted that the group had to be for kids, but I thought otherwise. When we walked into the room and found it filled with adults, some of whom had severe physical deformities from their scoliosis, I looked at my mother and said, "I told you so. No kids."

People shared their experiences with scoliosis that included practices no longer in effect. They spoke about medical issues that just did not pertain to me. I wished there were girls in braces to talk to so I could find out how they were dealing with this torture. I needed to find out how other girls my age talked about their scoliosis, how they wore their clothes, and how they dealt with wearing a brace in school and during the summer time. When we left the adult support group meeting, my mother admitted that I was right. I hated my brace and how it altered my life.

> Why wasn't there an outlet where kids like me could express their frustration and pain?

"I wish they had a group like this with kids," I said to my mom.

My mother looked at me, and I could just tell that the wheels were turning under her crazy, curly black hair. "Leah, if you want, you can make your own group." And that is exactly what I proceeded to do.

I made up flyers and brought them to my orthopedist and physical therapy offices. I wanted to create an environment for girls like me who could comfortably display their braces without being judged. I needed to give voice to those who felt as I did, alone.

On August 6th, 2006, a few weeks before my 14th birthday, the Curvy Girls Scoliosis Support Group was born. Four girls attended the first meeting. We talked about school, clothes, friends, and other problems relating to our braces. I closed the group that day with a simple yet poignant message, "We all have something to deal with that will shape who we are to become; this is ours." This is a message that I try to live by every day.

Since that first meeting, we've held monthly meetings, with typically ten to fifteen girls attending. The mission of my group is to help girls not feel the loneliness I felt and to be able to learn from each other. I want them to have access to the support that I lacked. We raise awareness in schools and in our communities, fundraise, make hospital visits, support each other through texting and phone calls, shop for brace-friendly clothing, and provide support to girls all over the world on our website. I help other girls talk about their experiences with scoliosis.

I started the group because it felt right to me. It was a simple action and I never realized how much I would be able to affect these girls. I opened my doors and my arms in order to talk to people who were going through the same situation. When strangers thank me, it's a strange feeling. It feels so surreal that I can make an impact simply by sharing my experiences. By sharing my negative experiences, I can help change theirs.

HIGH SCHOOL

I was in the ninth grade the first time I started taking my brace off during school without my parents knowing. It was such a cute outfit, and the brace really spoiled the look of it. Plus, I was in high school now! I wanted to be cool, not ... lumpy. So right before first period, I went into the locker room, quickly whipped it off and stuck it in my gym locker, but this time it would wait there for six hours. I remember a feeling of paranoia that day. What if within those couple of hours, all the work I'd done for the past two years got messed up? The worst was the thought that someone would discover it in the locker room and either vandalize it or give it to one of the coaches, and then my mom would find out what I had done. I also remember that no one looked at me any differently that day. Maybe I wanted a couple of people to comment on how much better I looked without the brace. When it came down to it, I guess I realized how much people really couldn't tell when I was wearing it. I only did that a couple more times because each time I had the same gnawing feeling.

SO CLOSE

We always came back to Dr. Mermelstein; we trusted him. He always explained things so that we all understood. At one of my quarterly visits, he said we could probably start talking about weaning me off of the brace in a few months. It was the best news ever! As we left the examining room, we recognized a girl we met before, Julie. She and her mom were visibly upset. They had just been told that she would have to have surgery. While her body had grown and changed, her brace remained on the floor of her closet. I asked Julie to come to our support group. As we left, my mom and I discussed how lucky I was. And then, suddenly, my "luck" changed.

Only a couple of weeks after that appointment, I noticed that the sides of my waist were no longer symmetrical. We thought it might be caused by the brace pressing in on one side more than the other. Maybe it would look different when I was out of the brace for a couple of hours. After two hours of dance class without wearing my brace, I looked in the mirror and there it was—my asymmetrical waist. We made another appointment with Dr. Mermelstein, and instead of weaning me off the brace, this time the topic was surgery. Surgery. Yet I still had to wear my brace! I left that appointment and I was done.

When I found out that I had to have surgery after wearing the brace for two years, I just lost it. I cried a lot. It felt like I had no control over what was going on with my body anymore, and I didn't like that loss of control. My mom and I proceeded to fight about it.

She wanted me to continue wearing the brace, "just in case," but I was done. That night, I hid my brace in the boiler room and went off to school for the first time in two years without it. I had struggled for long enough and I just couldn't deal with it any longer. I had to make my own decision. In fact, I made a list that day at school called, "*10 Reasons I Don't Want To Wear My Brace.*" I remember showing it to my friends and having them read it before I presented it to my mom. I—Was—Done.

But what about the group? Was I going to have to stop leading the group? I wondered how I could help them now. Wasn't the goal to avoid surgery? Had I failed? How would I be able to sit in a room of Curvy Girls, and tell them that they need to keep wearing their braces? It didn't make sense until I realized that the group was about more than just what I said to the girls; it was about being surrounded by people feeling, saying, and going through the same experiences. Even if I'm not the perfect role model for the girls, I still have things to tell them that I wish people had told me. The bottom line is that I was alone for the beginning of my bracing years, and I didn't want any other girls to have to wake up dreading getting dressed and going through school the way that I had. No one should ever have to feel this way.

THE LAST STRAW

It was probably the first time I actually wanted to go to school. I was so done with doctor's appointments and second opinions, third opinions— and even fourth opinions—that I was literally using school as an excuse to not have to go to this "one last opinion" all the way in Brooklyn. I refused to get out of bed and into the car, so they did the only logical thing they had left to do: My gentle and generally supportive dad dragged me out of bed, hair a mess, no make-up, no glasses, and wearing raggedy pajamas. They threw me into the car, and off we went.

Before I knew it, I was sitting in the waiting room. All of these places look the same: magazines, gray walls, a couple of tattered children's books, and that toy with the different colored wires and beads. My mom was sitting next to me filling out the typical paperwork for the millionth time. It was the usual: name, d.o.b., insurance, blah, blah, blah. The silence was broken as she remarked, "It asks here, 'Have you ever been depressed?'" I didn't even look at her when the words emerged from my mouth, "Shut up." To which she responded in that stupidly sickening and obviously fake tone, "We don't talk like that. People don't want to hear that."

I was in shock. How could she really think I could care? She was fully aware that I'd rather be anywhere else than in yet another doctor's office, and I really couldn't have cared what other people might want at this point. After all, I was sitting there in my pajamas. Did I look like a person who cared? I was so tired of it all.

SURGERY

I had surgery June 29, 2007. As I am not one to sit still, surgery changed my lifestyle when they told me I couldn't do much physical activity for nine months to a year. Although I couldn't participate, I sat in on my dance classes and watched. It was pure torture. Instead of giving up my passions, I tried even harder. Once I was cleared to return to activities, I had to relearn how to do certain things, such as a rolling dance move or my golf swing. Not only was I weak, but my back—held together with rods and screws—was no longer familiar to me. Movement was restricted and limited. But I was determined. I took more dance classes, worked out at the gym, and did everything I could to reach my full potential. At my dance recital the following year, I performed in five challenging dance routines and was awarded Student of the Year at the dance studio I had attended since I was two and a half. My family was amazed. They remarked on how I became a better dancer now than before my surgery.

The main effect scoliosis has had on me is learning that no matter how big the setback, when I feel passionate about something and work hard enough, it can be done.

"Speech! Speech! Speech!" The 2,000-plus people in the crowd roared. I grasped the microphone in my shaking hand to make a speech I never would have imagined making. I looked over to see some of the Curvy Girls who were in the audience.

"I want to thank them. They have become such a huge part of my life and I have seen so many of them grow in so many different ways. As much as they come up to me saying thank you after every meeting, what they don't understand is, how grateful I am to them."

COMING FULL CIRCLE

My scoliosis has been a journey and a struggle, with life lessons learned. Looking back, there's no doubt in my mind that the brace helped me become the person I am today. I have learned to embrace standing out, as I unwittingly became comfortable with my individuality. I have developed confidence to speak up, even if my ideas may not be readily accepted. My voice, once stifled by my brace, now reverberates with a message of hope and perseverance. What began as a self-help group for local teens has developed into a humanistic mission that has touched the lives of teenagers across the country, and maybe around the world.

As a result of the publicity following the TeenNick HALO Awards, we opened our website curvygirlsscoliosis.com and Curvy Girls began to grow exponentially, both in the number of girls and families who joined our local group, as well as expanding nationally. No sooner did the show air, kids of all ages began to contact me asking how they could start a Curvy Girls' group in their area. We guide them through the process.

My mom doesn't want the girls to feel alone and I never want anyone to feel as I did.

After a few months, girls with scoliosis from all over the world began posting their own stories on our website. But you know what amazes me the most? Every girl, no matter where she is from, says the same things, has the same worries and concerns, yet feels alone because she can't find anyone else to relate to.

Curvy Girls' chapters are changing that one girl, one group, at a time.

Over the years I have been asked a variety of questions and thought this was the perfect platform to share the answers to many of them.

How much has Curvy Girls Scoliosis chapters grown since the writing of Straight Talk's first edition?

When the first book was published, there were 37 Curvy Girls' chapters. Now, we have more than 100 groups in almost all 50 states and are represented on each continent, with the exception of Antarctica, of course! But it's so much more than just the number of chapters. Curvy Girls has become synonymous with the scoliosis journey.

We've had four international conventions with hundreds of attendees. We've also set up a mentorship program, consisting of former CG Leaders, for our leaders to gain support and to further their leadership skills. The organization has evolved to be bigger than I ever could have imagined.

Curvy Girls has touched so many lives and is becoming pivotal in improving patient care. What means the most to me is when medical professionals know to recommend their local Curvy Girls' chapter to a newly diagnosed patient. To me, that indicates that medical professionals are recognizing the importance of mental health and how it can impact one's overall health.

Was it hard to decide not to have boys in the support group?

When starting out I just wanted to talk to anyone who was wearing a brace; it didn't matter who! But it turned out that three girls showed up for the first meeting and it was only girls who kept coming back. We determined it would be best to have meetings for only those who identified as girls. We wanted to preserve the dynamic of the group. There are many things that girls are likely to not feel comfortable talking about in front of boys, such as wearing a bra with a brace or getting your period, which is an important indicator of growth that we want to be able to celebrate.

We believe that keeping meetings for only those identifying as girls makes it a more comfortable space for the group as a whole. However, we encourage all of our leaders and members to support everyone they meet going through scoliosis! And we hope that some of the information and tips that are offered in Straight Talk are shared no matter a person's gender.

How many years has it been since you've had surgery?

I had my surgery in June 2007. Based on when you're reading this book, you'll have to do the math on that one!

Were you upset when you found out you needed surgery after wearing your brace for almost three years?

Upset is just one of many emotions I felt. I was upset at the prospect of how my life might change. I also felt scared, because the idea of a big surgery is intimidating. There was a little feeling of relief—I had this feeling that my scoliosis would be "fixed," and I wouldn't have to worry about my spine. As I got older, I, of course, learned that there's no such thing as "fixing" scoliosis; I still have scoliosis. And then I also felt just generally anxious about all of the unknowns.

Remember, there are no wrong or normal feelings to experience when you get big news like that.

Did you ever learn the Schroth Method?

I just recently learned it! Yes, over a decade after being braced and many years after getting surgery, I decided to reach out to my local Schroth therapist. It was a decision I made because I wanted to be sure I was moving correctly when working out and going about my everyday life. I was at a point where I knew I'd be able to commit to it and incorporate it into my daily routine. It's not too late to take action if you're feeling the same way.

Have you ever had pain over the years after surgery?

No, but I've had some discomforts. Especially if I'm not active for a while or if I'm sitting for too long, particularly in a car or on a plane. This is where these excercises plays a big part.

Have you made any changes in your lifestyle to maintain the health of your spine?

In college I got into running and even ran a half marathon! But I knew it wasn't an activity I should continue long-term. Because of where I'm fused (T5-L4), I learned that I only have a few vertebrae absorbing the impact of running. Because I need to protect those vertebrae, running wasn't a good long-term activity. So, I've found other ways to stay active while protecting my spine, like biking and hiking. If I'm in the gym, I'll opt for the elliptical, bike, or stair climber, rather than the treadmill. I also play a lot of golf, and between you and me, I think having a fused spine makes my golf swing even better.

Do you think it's important for girls to learn Physical Therapy Scoliosis-Specific Exercises (PSSE), such as the Schroth Method, if they are fused?

Yes! Something that was explained to me is that the surgery "fixes" your spine, but it's not doing anything for your muscles. You have to take that into your own hands. In essence, the muscles in your back have spent years in one position and after surgery, they're going to stay like that unless you work to lengthen and strengthen them. For example, you might still feel more tightness or flexibility on one side over the other in your neck or hips. This is where Schroth comes in. Your therapist will help you understand your muscles and how to make small adjustments specific to your curve. It might sound similar to a yoga instructor, but remember, these therapists are specifically trained and certified to understand scoliosis. Overall, I feel that learning Schroth is really empowering for one's long-term physical health.

I saw you've done some work with international model Martha Hunt. Can you tell me more about that?

Martha Hunt reached out to Curvy Girls in 2017 with a beautiful idea to create a piece of jewelry with Pluma Italia that would empower those with scoliosis, and she wanted to donate the proceeds to Curvy Girls. For Martha, scoliosis is personal—she had spinal fusion surgery when she was a teenager (Fun Fact: Her surgery was exactly 10 days before mine) and, just like a lot of you, said she never knew anyone with scoliosis prior to her surgery.

Martha designed the necklace to have "inégal" on one side, which is French for "uneven," and "resilient" on the other, a word she selected to encapsulate how we face our scoliosis journey.

We decided to name the necklace "Alyson" in honor of our mutual friend Alyson Gerber, author of *Braced*, who also has scoliosis, and inspires us with her story. Martha organized a photoshoot to launch the necklace, modeled by Curvy Girls, showing off their scoliosis. Teen Vogue was there to cover the day and publish a video and article about the photoshoot and necklace.

One of the coolest parts of the photoshoot was how adamant Martha was that she wanted the girls to be able to pick their own clothes, hair, and make-up. It was so important to her that each of the girls had a voice in how they looked and felt in front of the camera. Another standout memory was when, surrounded by over a dozen Curvy Girls, Martha shared that this was the most people with scoliosis she had ever met.

A year later, Martha designed a second piece of the Inégal jewelry line, a rose gold bracelet that she named Leah, one of my greatest honors.

Since our initial project, Martha has done so much for Curvy Girls, from being a co-MC at the Convention's Fashion Show, to shouting us out on countless interviews and videos. She's an incredible advocate for scoliosis and the organization. I am personally so grateful to her for sharing our mission. She has a lot more on the horizon to drive positive change in scoliosis treatment, so keep your eyes out for what's next!

How did you meet author Alyson Gerber?

Alyson reached out to me to read an advance copy of her book *Braced* and provide a quote for the back of the book. I absolutely devoured the book; I had never read a story where the main character spoke to the concerns and emotions that I felt at that time in my life. I was honored to provide a quote. When reading the "about the author" section, I learned she lived in Brooklyn and reached out to meet up for coffee. I had to know how much of the story was based on her own journey. She shared that the heart of the story and the emotions the main character feels are very similar to hers. It was incredible getting to learn how she translated her journey into a full-length book. We've been great friends ever since!

Where do you see Curvy Girls in 10 years?

World domination! What's most important to me is that I never want anyone to feel alone in their journey. It's so important for each of you to continue to share your story and to pass along the support you receive.

With that, I'd also like to take this time and thank all our families who are involved with Curvy Girls. I appreciate everyone's dedication to the Curvy Girls' mission and continued support over the years. This organization could never have grown and accomplished everything it has without each and every one of YOU!

WHERE LEAH IS TODAY

Today, Leah works in advertising in New York City. As President and Founder of Curvy Girls, Leah is still amazed by how much her little support group has grown to more than 100 group leaders internationally. She is grateful to all the chapter leaders and members who through the years have made the CG mission their own. Representing Curvy Girls at conferences and in interviews around the world, she is passionate about speaking on the power of peer support and urging medical professionals to connect patients with their local CG chapter.

Straight Talk Scoliosis — The Journey Continues

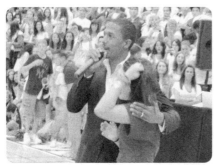

Nick Cannon announces, "I'm here to give back to someone who's been giving back her entire life."

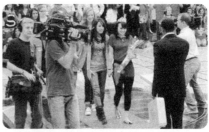

A tiara is placed on Leah's head and she is handed a bouquet of red roses before she walks the red carpet with fellow Curvy Girl Rachel Mulvaney.

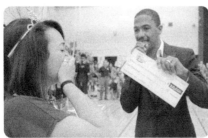

Nick Cannon hands Leah two checks — one for $10,000 for scoliosis research, and a second for $10,000 to help offset college expenses.

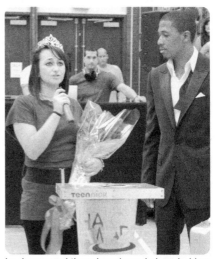

Leah grasped the microphone in her shaking hand to make a speech that she could never have imagined giving.

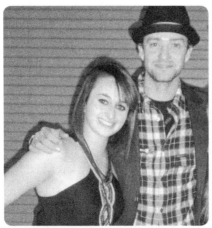

Justin Timberlake flies Leah back to Las Vegas, Nevada, for his Shriners Children's Hospital Benefit Concert.

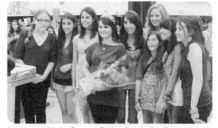

Leah and her Curvy Girls: Danielle Greenberg, Liv Mevorach, Alexis Bell, Leah Stoltz, Rachel Mulvaney, Victoria Smith, Esther Beck, Deanna Albro, and Jenna Stern.

Photo credits: Paige McCoy, Patrice Stern, Robin Stoltz

© 2012 Viacom International Inc. All rights reserved. Nickelodeon, TeenNick Halo Awards and all related titles, logos and characters are trademarks of Viacom International Inc.

Part 1: Memoirs

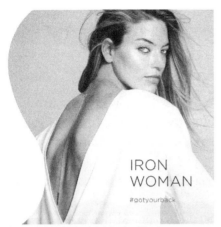
International Model, Martha Hunt

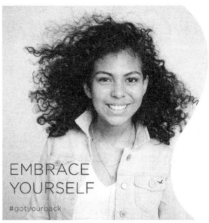
Melissa Serrano, New Jersey

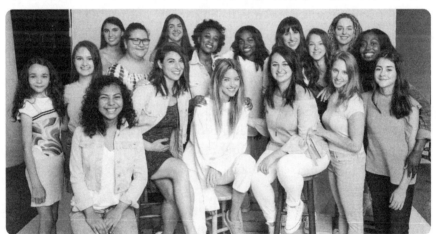
Group Photo: *Front Row L to R:* Melissa Serrano, Alyson Gerber, Martha Hunt, Leah Stoltz, Jenny Elf, Laura Garcia; *Back Row L to R:* Rebeca Hernandez, Julianne Martin, Gianna Calligy, Katie Thorn, Dana Keogler, Narissa Johnson, Kaalund Valerie, Rachel Mulvaney, Brielle Neumann, Nicole Agaronnik, Jamiah Bennett

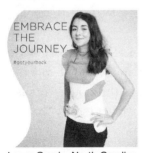
Laura Garcia, North Carolina

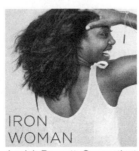
Jamiah Bennett, Connecticut

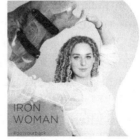
Nicole Agaronnik, New York

Photo credit: Jason McDonald

Adolescence or Scoliosis?

Robin

"Start the car. When I say 'go,' you drive." Those were my husband's instructions for the get-away. We thought we had a solid plan for getting our daughter, Leah, to the doctor's office for yet another scoliosis appointment. But it wasn't playing out the way we had hoped. The commotion upstairs continued, punctuated by wild screams of, "I'm not going anywhere."

Leah clutched her bed sheets as her father pulled her from the bed. Leah's rescue dog, Squirt, began to bark and jump in a vain effort to save his pal from her attacker. Arms flailing wildly only stayed by door jams in vain attempts to harness herself to the house. Her 200- pound once-gentle-and-kind father pried her fingers off while carrying her pajama-clad body screaming and crying down the steps and out the front door. With continued protests and a last-ditch attempt to brace herself on the car door, he loaded our once-sweet-and-compliant child into the back seat of the get-away car, along with the trailing bed sheets and random shoes.

Who is this child? No clothing other than pajamas. No eye glasses. No coat. It's cold in New York in February, but we're off. Only there's one problem.

In all the confusion, Leah's four-legged protector had jumped in alongside his charge. So now, huffing and puffing, her dad must remove the dog while somehow keeping our child in the car. She was either too busy kicking the back of my driver's seat to notice the opportunity for escape, or she was just too tired. Crouched down in the seat, she continued kicking and screaming well onto the Northern State Parkway and intermittently when she remembered.

What happened to our daughter? Normally, Leah didn't leave the house without her full accoutrements of make-up and well-put-together clothes. Not unlike many adolescent girls, leaving the house entails a solid hour of closet and mirror time. We would have bet money that she would have gotten herself dressed and ready as soon as we told her we would be taking her "as is." But as any parent of a teenager can tell you, during adolescence, all bets are off! Power struggling with a teenager is a lose-lose situation. Now, add scoliosis on top and you don't know if you are coming or going. Lose-lose lose-lose.

Leah had always been a happy and cooperative child, very inquisitive and interested in going places and experiencing new things. She willingly went to all the other physician's visits, consults, and orthotists. What happened?

This was our fourth consultation and she'd had enough, enough with visits to different doctors, and enough with braces. She'd had it with me for making these "random" appointments, and she'd had enough with feeling "different" than other girls her age. And now, she's afraid of what the future may hold. She's afraid that if she has surgery, she won't be able to do what she loves most, to dance.

"How long will I have to give up dance?" she asks at each consultation.

This is how a young teen makes a decision about which surgeon is right for her. She cries when the doctors, nurses, and physician assistants ask her about herself, and it breaks our hearts.

Leah was diagnosed with adolescent idiopathic scoliosis toward the end of the sixth grade, when she was eleven and a half years old. One evening while getting ready for bed, she came into my bedroom and said, "Feel this; my back feels weird." Leah was able to reach her arms all the way around and feel her own back. We thought she was just very flexible, but we later learned from the physical therapist that part of the problem was that she lacked stability. Was this a precursor for scoliosis? Was this the same reason her spine was too mobile? We are not aware of the definitive answer to these questions but the physical therapist believed this to be related.

Sure enough, as Leah instructed me to feel her back, I could feel a distinct curve as I ran my fingers along the upper part of her spine. Not only was I able to feel it, but now I clearly saw a curve I had never seen before. I wondered how the spine was able to bend like that; I thought the spinal column was supposed to be rigid and straight. I knew all the body's nerves ran through this area, so how was it that the spine could curve without causing a problem to the rest of the body? Maybe it was denial, the defense mechanism that runs interference for our psyche when experiencing something difficult. In my lame attempt to make sense of and normalize what I was feeling, I thought about the crown of a baby's head and how their skull bones move together as the baby grows. This must be the same type of process that happens before entering adolescence. I figured that as soon as the body caught up to the spine, the spinal column would surely straighten.

At her annual check-up that weekend, we pointed out our concerns about Leah's spine. The pediatrician said that while it wasn't significant, we could see an orthopedist if I was concerned. I made an appointment for the next day.

Upon examining Leah, the orthopedist also initially thought the curve was minor (approximately 15°), but the X-rays showed otherwise. Leah hid her curve "nicely." Not only wasn't it obvious to the untrained eye, it apparently wasn't visible to the trained eye. Leah's scoliosis was completely missed during the school scoliosis screening only five months prior. X-rays revealed that her primary curve was 37°, with a secondary compensatory curve of 26°. She gave the appearance of being balanced because her top and bottom were twisted in opposing directions.

At the time of Leah's diagnosis and bracing, my husband, Mike, was in the hospital under quarantine for radioactive treatment of thyroid cancer. He didn't even know Leah had been diagnosed with scoliosis because there was no way to reach him. I remember Dr. Mermelstein's calm and kindness; he was just like Leah's dad who never panicked. He was reassuring and direct while he explained the course of treatment for a 37° curve.

Later that same day, Leah was fitted for a back brace that she would work up to wearing twenty-two hours a day, seven days a week for a yet to-be-determined period of time. Her Risser measured zero at bracing, which meant that her growth plates were fully open. The trick now was to keep her spine from further curving while her growth continued. This posed an ironic twist for a mother: wanting your child to grow quickly, at a time when what I also wanted was to hold onto the innocence of her childhood. I felt as if I was being cheated.

Leah appeared to take this new information in stride. When we picked up her new brace the following week, I watched for her expression. She didn't seem upset so I kept my demeanor calm. I didn't want to alarm her to the strangeness of what I was seeing: a large plastic contraption that she would have to put around her developing body for two years! I couldn't fathom how she would be able to do this. The whole concept seemed archaic to me. Thoughts ran through my mind, "How would she ever wear something so large? Was she really going to agree to wear it? Maybe she should just skip to the surgery since that is where this may end up anyway." It seemed insurmountable, but since kids tend to follow their parents' lead, I thought it best to keep my own feelings in check and watch for her reaction. She would have enough of her own feelings to deal with; she shouldn't have to take on mine.

BRACE REALITY

It wasn't until two days after we picked up the brace that I heard Leah crying in her room. She couldn't find anything to wear that fit over her brace. We would have to go shopping. When she couldn't even find something to wear to go shopping, her crying and sense of despair grew. She cried that she just wanted to have the surgery. I couldn't imagine how we were going to find stylish clothes to go over this contraption. My heart sunk inside for her. Because kids at her age are influenced by what their peers think, my biggest worry was that someone would say something to embarrass her and she wouldn't know how to respond. I prayed she had the strength to know that the brace did not define her.

We made up scenarios about what she could say if someone asked about her brace. She only had one week of school remaining before summer vacation. She'd have the whole summer to get used to it. I wanted her to feel stronger about herself before she had to face her peers. Initially, Leah tried her best to disguise her brace but would eventually find that the best way to deal with it was to come right out and talk about it. This way, there was no secret worry about being caught off guard.

I have a coping strategy that helps me keep perspective when I feel overwhelmed. I tell myself, "Short of life-threatening, I can deal with anything." I couldn't fix what was happening to Leah. I couldn't stop it or protect her from the reality of it, but what I *could* do was support her and help her to develop strength; strength that could serve her through life's many challenges. I learned from my own childhood challenges and in my profession from my clients, that it is the resilience of a person that counts the most in the face of adversity. We are always faced with challenges, but if we teach our children that they can bounce back, we give them a sense of confidence and self-reliance. Leah says it best when she tells Curvy Girls, "Everyone has something they have to deal with, and this is ours."

SQUIRT

When Mike and I saw how diligent Leah was with wearing and taking care of her brace, we rewarded her with a long-awaited dog. Well, he wasn't exactly the puppy that Leah had in mind when they ventured off on their search, but Mike knew that this nervous, depressed dog needed a home. Squirt attached himself to Leah and only Leah. He would wait by her bedroom door all day for her to return home from school. He even had a crooked tail, just like her back.

Leah wore her brace faithfully for the first year, yet her main curve increased by ten degrees, measuring at 47°. Because the change was gradual, taking place over a year's time, our orthopedist was not concerned. We would wait and see if it stabilized. Over the following year, it did indeed stabilize at around the 50° point, and cosmetically she still did not look compromised. Leah didn't have the typical shoulder protrusion, which was the telltale sign of scoliosis. She looked balanced, and her body hid her curve.

ADOLESCENCE + SCOLIOSIS = ?

As time progressed, so did adolescence. While we were in the thick of things, it was difficult to distinguish between adolescent defiance and frustration with having to wear a body brace. The ramifications of scoliosis seemed to propel her full force into adolescent angst.

She stopped hugging me. Leah seemed angry with me all the time. That is, until Sunday when it was time for our support group and her whole demeanor towards me would change. During a joint parent-teen Curvy Girls' group session, she sat herself on my lap and related to me as if she did this all the time. Somehow it was safe. She was in control of her life on those Sundays, and not the victim to her scoliosis. When the meeting ended, she'd return to her pattern of feigned indifference until the following month.

Quietly, she tortured herself, hiding her thoughts and feelings behind a facade of indifference. One day after a night of nasty fighting, I picked Leah up from school and asked her how she felt about the night before. Her response was, in no uncertain terms, "I don't do feelings." Ah, yes, why would she "do feelings" when both her dad and I are social workers. That is what we "do" for a living—feelings. What better way to separate and establish her own identity but to not "do" what we "do." And so her conundrum: Share my feelings with my parents or stuff my feelings and pretend that I don't care.

END IN SIGHT

At our two-year check-up, the orthopedist said we could anticipate a plan for brace weaning at the next visit. With relief and celebration, we readied to leave the office, when we spotted another fourteen-year-old girl and her mother. Their expressions were not the same as ours. The girl's eyes were red from crying and the mother looked stunned. Their news was quite different. Leah and I stayed to talk with them. We offered comfort, and exchanged phone numbers and email addresses. Her surgery was scheduled to be in three months. Leah invited her to the support group, and Julie came with her mother. When we left the office, I told Leah, "There by the grace of God, go us." You just never know. But Leah reminded me, "She didn't wear her brace." She hated it and refused to wear it. It sat on the floor of her closet.

Well, that made sense. The formula was simple:

Wear your brace = no surgery. Don't wear it = surgery.

Or so we thought, until two weeks later.

"My waist is not even," Leah exclaimed.

(Again, denial.) "Maybe, it's from the brace," I responded.

Two days later, after being out of her brace for two hours while in dance, Leah again pointed out, "Look at it now." There it was, plain to see. One side of her waist was almost perfectly straight, while the other showed what I thought must be her newly developing waistline.

Within a few days' time, back to the orthopedist we went. This time we were not as lucky. As he studied her waist, we realized it was the defining moment. Because her curve was in the lumbar region of her body, when her body developed and her waist slimmed, the scoliosis showed itself.

After two-plus years of wearing her brace, Leah was told she needed surgery. Listening to your child sob "Why me?" alone in her bedroom was heart-wrenching. Leah would have her brace/scoliosis meltdowns periodically, usually in the shower. Ultimately, she would emerge relieved. This time I could hear her dog, Squirt, whimpering outside the bathroom door. When I got closer, I could hear her angry sobs, "I wore my brace for nothing."

Leah's acting out became almost unbearable once she knew that she needed surgery. She was angry and felt as if the years spent in a brace were for naught, even though wearing the brace for those two critical years ultimately enabled her to have a better surgical outcome.

Leah saw surgery as a personal failure. She wondered how she could lead the group when she had "failed." In her mind her body had failed her and she would now fail the group of girls she wanted to support. She was surprised when I reminded her that the support group she began was not just about her giving to others. Other people needed to be able to give to her as well, to be able to offer her what she had given them. She didn't have to be the strong one or have all the answers all the time; she, too, could cry and feel scared. She seemed satisfied and continued with the group.

The last Curvy Girls' group meeting before Leah's surgery was not held at our house, as it usually was. Instead, Curvy Girl Rachel Mulvaney with her mom, Terry, wanted us to be guests at their home. They wanted to thank Leah for all that she had done. They celebrated Leah that day. The girls bought Leah gifts useful for her hospital stay. There were fun colored leg rolls and soft coughing pillows for after surgery, a journal to keep track of the "f" word (feelings). When I left that day, I too, had learned the true meaning of support.

From the very onset, we felt confident with our orthopedist. But when it came time for surgery, we worried about where we should have it done. We were too close to Manhattan, with some of the best medical facilities in the world, not to consider the options there. Mike and I kept saying, "You don't know what you don't know." We had to go and find out everything we didn't know, so we could feel like we knew even less. Our search into The City began. At our first encounter with "The Office with the Attitude," we were told surgery is done at 40° and the oh-so-sensitive physician assistant proceeded to tell Leah that the brace she wore for two years was "useless" compared to the one that they make. Great message!

Then we had another consult with a surgeon who authored one of the few books written on scoliosis. What was most baffling was the difference in "expert" opinions. Each one had something different to say, which accounted for the final crazy-parent-drags-pajama-clad-child-to-Brooklyn visit. Our final and last consult was more consistent with what we heard from our own orthopedist. How were we to make sense of all the information? Should we have surgery? If so, when and with whom?

In the end, it was our own orthopedist who helped us sort through all the information we gathered and make sense of the differing opinions. He spent a couple of hours with us after the office closed, sitting at the computer, showing X-rays of varying surgical procedures, teaching, and answering every last one of our questions. He taught us that sometimes medicine is more of an art than a science. When we left, we knew he was to be our artist. He is brilliant, talented, and kind, and he leaves his ego at the door. Ultimately, the time Leah spent with Dr. Mermelstein helped her come to terms with having surgery sooner rather than later.

The local Long Island facility where Leah had surgery, Good Samaritan Hospital, was a superior experience, a gem in our own backyard. When all was said and done, Leah was happy with the outcome of her surgery. She is pleased with how her body looks and proud of the scar that runs almost the full length of her back. The first day back to school after surgery, she wore a halter-top that her dad thought too revealing. But we decided that if she was willing to "expose" her scar, she could wear that shirt. She returned to dance much sooner than she thought and now her behavior is relatively normal. That is to say, if you consider adolescence a time of normalcy!

Leah has since finished her bracing, and surgery is literally "behind" her. As a young adult, she has taken to working through issues related to how wearing a back brace and having major spine surgery made her feel about her body. Along the way, Leah learned that she wasn't alone, that she could positively impact her own life circumstances, could speak up for herself—and teach others to do the same. Perhaps more importantly, she learned that she could take control over her own body and assert herself even in uncomfortable situations. Scoliosis presented her with challenges but afforded her these many gifts.

Rachel

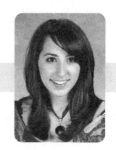

Meet Rachel from Long Island

Age: 14

Braced at age 11

Rachel enjoys drawing and painting. She also appreciates spending time with her friends and family, and watching old Hollywood films.

Rachel's goal is to give back what she was given—the ability to listen while helping others with the challenges presented by scoliosis.

Rachel's experience has taught her the meaning of determination. She challenged herself to do whatever she could to exceed her perceived limitations in order to keep her scoliosis at bay. She too wore her brace faithfully for two and a half years, yet when she was finally brace-free, her curve continued to progress. Her commitment and success turned her fears into setting and achieving her goals, while allowing this strength of determination to fuel her.

Rachel's Message: It's never too late to take back control over your body.

Rachel Mulvaney and her mother, Terry Mulvaney

I Wouldn't Change a Thing

SCHOOL SCREENING

Rachel: I was nine years old, and in the third grade, when my class was called down to the nurse's office for a scoliosis test. I watched as five or six kids ahead of me got tested. The only thing they had to do was lift up their shirt, bend forward, and leave with a lollipop, which put a smile on everyone's face. Unlike them, I left with a puzzled face because my exam was strangely different. Once my shirt was lifted and I bent forward, the nurse gasped. I had no idea what was going on. The doctor asked me to stand up straight, bend forward again, rotate to the left, and then to the right. He examined my back by feeling the direction of my spinal column. I was then asked to sit back down and let the rest of the class finish their scoliosis test. After my second examination, the nurse handed me a note to give to my mom. I didn't have the slightest clue at that time as to the challenges I would soon face. When I got home that day, I gave my mom the note and she too lifted up my shirt. It was a relief to not hear a gasp come from her.

Mom: Rachel is my fourth and last child, and this was the first-time scoliosis was introduced to my family as a possible threat. I had little understanding of this condition, which is why I felt uncomfortable receiving a call from Rachel's school nurse that she failed her scoliosis screening. With a touch of sensitive concern in her voice, she advised me to make an appointment with the pediatrician as soon as possible to either confirm or deny the school's findings.

I immediately called my pediatrician's office, and in the middle of my unusually long explanation as to why I needed an appointment as soon as possible, the office assistant interjected, "The school nurses are never right. We get kids all the time who fail the school scoliosis screening and pass our evaluation. There's absolutely no need to worry." I was comforted by her words, so we set an appointment for the following week. When Rachel came home she presented me with the nurse's notice; I immediately felt a twinge of anxiety.

"Rachel, can I see your back?" I asked her. Without hesitation, she lifted the back of her shirt and bent over. I stared at her back and ran my fingers up and down her spine for some time, trying to see or feel a curve, but her back seemed straight to me. My own observations, plus the comment from the assistant in the pediatrician's office, prompted me to think that this was just some miscalculation that would be corrected in a week.

On the day of the appointment, I was calm and confident. This was just a formality that would be over in a few minutes, and then we would go on as if nothing happened. My state of mind quickly changed after the pediatrician confirmed the school's findings. "Rachel has a curve of about 15°, and she should immediately see a pediatric orthopedic physician specializing in scoliosis." I went from blissful ignorance to panic.

I repeated silently to myself, "What did that mean?" As I stumbled with my thoughts, I knew I needed to pull myself together and start asking questions.

"What does it mean that her curve is 15°? Is that serious? What is a normal curve?"

The physician responded, "A curve that is 0° to 10° is considered to be within the normal range." "Okay, that's not too bad; she's only off by 5°," I thought.

The doctor then asked, "Has Rachel begun to menstruate?"

I was taken aback. I could not understand why Rachel's menstruation was a matter for questioning at that moment. It was as though the doctor read my mind and immediately continued, "Girls will continue to grow for twelve- to eighteen-months after they begin to menstruate. A close monitoring will be necessary since Rachel has years left of growth."

By the end of our visit, we scheduled a consultation with an orthopedic specialist. Determined to be better prepared for the next appointment I decided to give myself a quick education about this condition through the internet. Within seconds my computer screen was instantly flooded with all kinds of images and information. I was not ready or prepared to see such severe scoliosis cases. Emotionally drained, I closed the web page and decided to get educated by the professionals, and not the internet.

MEETING THE LOLLIPOP DOCTOR

Rachel: The first time I met my orthopedic doctor I liked her. She made a great first impression, as she greeted me with a handful of colorful lollipops for me to choose from. She made talking to her very easy. She asked me a series of questions such as, "How do you like school?" and "What kinds of activities do you like to do?" I told her all about my teachers and how much I loved to dance. She also lifted up my shirt and kept admiring how flexible I was. We were told to come back in six months for new X-rays.

Mom: Rachel's orthopedic physician was younger than we expected, warm, and very friendly. More importantly, I could tell that Rachel was comfortable because she was quickly engaged in conversation with her. Impressed with Rachel's flexibility, she encouraged her to continue to be physically active, as this would help with her condition. She confirmed that Rachel had idiopathic scoliosis with a curve of 16°; however, we were relieved to learn that no treatment was required unless her curve approached the 25° mark. In order to monitor the progression of the curve, Rachel needed to come back in six months for a follow-up visit and a new set of X-rays. Unfortunately, when we returned for this appointment, we learned that the doctor's office no longer accepted our medical insurance. We did our best to challenge their information, but were unsuccessful. The receptionist apologized for the miscommunication; they were under the impression that we had been contacted. The next day I began my search for a new orthopedic physician.

Several weeks later, I found a new doctor in our health plan; however, his first appointment wasn't for six months, which would have made Rachel's follow-up a full year later. Determined to get an earlier appointment with another specialist, I declined. This turned out to be a decision I would later regret. Unconsciously, I was allowing Rachel's scoliosis to take the back burner while I let other seemingly more serious problems take priority in our lives.

STRUGGLING WITH LIFE'S DEMAND

Rachel: During this time there was a lot going on with my family. We moved into a new house, I went to a new school, and my grandfather became very sick. Within six months of moving, my grandfather, who I was very close to, passed away on my sister's birthday. It was the saddest day of my life and it seemed to only get worse. Six weeks later, our dog, Honey, had unexpectedly died. Nothing seemed to be going right. I tried to tell my mom I had back pain, but I could tell she wasn't taking what I said seriously. It was as if there was a black cloud over our family. My grandmother was depressed from losing her husband, and my sister was out of school for nearly three months with a severe case of mononucleosis. My back pain persisted, but I kept it to myself. I didn't want to add more stress onto my mom.

One evening, my pain became too obvious to hide. I couldn't walk without discomfort and I finally asked my mom to rub my back. It was then she realized that the pain I had complained about was real.

Mom: It felt as if a thousand things were happening at once. Up until Rachel's diagnosis, life might have been crazy, but somehow, I was able to balance it all. Then, in an instant, everything changed. The six months following the death of my father was an emphatic testament of the old saying, "When it rains, it pours." It was during this period when Rachel began to complain of back pain. As horrible as it sounds, I couldn't deal with it, not after losing my dad and having to face a long list of adversities that seemed to pile up aggressively against my family. I am embarrassed to admit that I ignored my daughter's complaints, convincing myself that her back pain was no big deal, and that she just wanted attention.

It wasn't until weeks later that I noticed she was bent forward holding her left hand on her lower back. She looked up at me and said that her back was killing her, could I please rub it. I motioned her to come over to me and she lay forward on my lap. I was dumbfounded as I pulled her top up, and frightened at what I saw.

The lower left side protruded like a small hump, while the right side of her back appeared normal. While I continued to rub her back, I couldn't help but notice an unmistakable bend in her spinal column that pulled to her right. The entire right side of her back seemed to bulge out. Her right rib cage protruded and appeared disproportionate to the other side. The center and left side appeared to be sunken in comparison to the protruding side. I felt physically sick as I realized that this child was not seeking attention; she was in pain. I felt like the world's worst mother.

The next day I made an appointment with the first office I took Rachel to. The office manager and I were able to arrange a payment plan that was affordable.

THE TURTLE SHELL

Rachel: The next thing I knew, I was back to see the "Lollipop Doctor." I'm not sure how, but there we were a year and a half later back where it all started. It was at this office visit that we learned my curve had gone from 16° to 35°. I heard the doctor tell my mom that I needed to be braced immediately. She further explained that I had to wear this back brace for sixteen hours a day for the next two- to three-years. I thought she was crazy, especially when she started to describe what the brace looked like, and how it would fit my body.

"It's like being in a very tight turtle shell," the doctor said.

I couldn't help but cry. I remember my mother just holding me and saying, "Rachel you can do this. Don't cry. Everything will be okay."

Mom: My eyes swelled with tears and my lips began to quiver, as I silently began to blame myself for this entire mess I put my daughter in. I tried to speak without breaking down, as I watched Rachel try to process what all of this meant. In a very shaky voice, I managed to ask, "How can your estimation be either two or three years?"

"Well, I don't know for sure, it depends on how much growing she has left to do. She hasn't begun to menstruate, and the growth plate in her pelvis is at a zero," she explained.

"Okay, well what number will tell you that she's done growing?"

"When she reaches a Risser 5, her growing is complete. This concerns me because we usually discuss corrective surgery when her curve hits the 40° mark," she concluded.

A million things were rushing through my mind, but the most important was figuring out a way to help Rachel get through whatever might lie ahead. Before we left, we were given a list of prosthetic offices that made the Boston Brace. On the way home, Rachel began to cry uncontrollably and I tried to hide the tears rolling down my face.

LET'S STRAP THEM IN

Rachel: Within forty-eight hours, I was being fitted for my first brace—the worst experience of my life. I never knew a medical professional could be so rude and inconsiderate of a child's pain. I was hysterical crying and he never once asked, "What's the matter?" It was my mother who asked, "Why is she crying like this?"

His answer was, "She's not used to wearing a brace yet." I gave him a dirty look and said, "No, I feel like I can't breathe. Please take it off!" More tears came down my cheeks and I said again, "Take it off!"

And all he said to me was, "Suck in your stomach and hold your breath," as he yanked each strap as tight as possible.

Mom: Having my child fitted for a back brace for the first time by a local orthotist was extremely foreign to me. I knew nothing about this process. The orthotist warned me how much my child would cry and complain regarding the discomfort of the brace. This translated to mean that I needed to be especially strong. I reminded myself that if Rachel was sick and had to take a horrible tasting medication in order to get well—even if she cried, I would make sure she would take it. I watched as they roughly maneuvered her, measured, and prodded her with their instruments. No matter how strong I told myself I had to be, my heart was breaking watching Rachel's eyes well up with tears. At one point they put the brace on so tight that Rachel immediately began to cry. It was the worst feeling in the world because I felt like I wasn't allowed to say anything. And to be completely honest, I was scared and too intimidated to speak up.

Rachel: I couldn't wait to get out of that office, and when we left, I ripped the straps right off. Finally, I could breathe. I thought these people were out of their minds to think I'm going to wear this contraption for sixteen hours a day.

> I think every doctor in the field of scoliosis should be fitted for a back brace and wear it for one week.

What better way to understand what it feels like to be strapped and pulled so tight, like a boa constrictor holding its prey.

My parents kept saying that everything would be okay, but the only thought I had was "easier said than done."No one knew the emotional and physical pain I was going through, let alone how scared and alone I truly felt.

All I kept doing was going over everything in my head. My mind was filled with anger, fear, and frustration. I was angry that I had to wear this horrible brace, scared that I might not be able to find clothes to hide this brace from the world, and frustrated because there were no guarantees. You see, I could do everything they told me, and still have to face surgery one day. They just didn't get it.

Mom: The next day we met back at the doctor's office for another set of X-rays, but this time she was to be X-rayed wearing the brace in order to see how well the brace was correcting her curve. She measured 35° without a brace, and 25° with the brace on. Again, not ever thinking to question the professional, I believed this was good; the brace was doing its job no matter what discomfort Rachel was experiencing. Wrong. I would later learn that bracing shouldn't cause that much pain.

As the weeks progressed, so did Rachel's pain. I continued to bring her back to the doctor, and though they never called her a liar, they reminded me that scoliosis does not cause pain. I knew my daughter wasn't lying. If she said she was in pain, then she was in pain. They gave her anti-inflammatory medications, but that didn't work. They ordered an MRI but that could not be completed, because no one realized that Rachel's orthodontic braces created a terrible pulling sensation as the magnets in the machine traveled further towards her upper body. My frustrations only escalated. I wasn't sure whom to be angrier with, her doctor who ordered the test, or the technician who clearly did not read that there was metal in her mouth.

BEING POWERLESS

Rachel: To be honest, I think the hardest part of the entire journey was just feeling angry all the time. I hated how this feeling took control of me. Whenever my mom tried to say something supportive, I didn't want to hear it; I didn't care. She didn't get it, no one did. Everything was changing so quickly in my life and I felt like I had no control. I was totally powerless.

To make matters worse, I learned that my father allowed my teacher to tell my entire class that I had scoliosis and that I would have to wear a back brace to school every day. What was my dad thinking, or my teacher? Why would they believe that kids in the fifth grade would be mature enough to handle my diagnosis of scoliosis? I guess now I realize they were trying to help, but I wish someone back then had asked me my opinion.

Every day, wearing this brace to school became harder because everyone knew. Everyone wanted to see it, touch it, and yes, some of the girls wanted to try it on. I was so angry at my mom for making me wear this stupid brace to school. She would say she understood, but she didn't. She wasn't living, breathing, eating, or sleeping in this thing—I was.

Mom: When no answers were found, I observed my once active outgoing daughter become very withdrawn, no longer going out or interacting with her friends. Since we were just bracing after school in the beginning, she would literally come home, do her homework, and then go to sleep on either the couch or her bed for hours. When this routine of hers continued for weeks, I called my pediatrician's office for an exam. I truly began to fear that Rachel had a serious medical condition since she was so lethargic. The pediatrician listened to the symptoms and then asked Rachel if there been any recent changes in her life. She mentioned that her grandfather died, we had lost our family dog, and that she just found out she has to wear this brace for sixteen hours a day (which she demonstrated by knocking on her stomach) because of her scoliosis.

The doctor then asked Rachel, "How's the bracing going?"

Rachel responded in a low, fragile voice, "Okay, I guess."

He began to ask more questions and we soon learned that years ago his daughter was also diagnosed with scoliosis. This seemed to help Rachel open up, and I began to hear all the emotional and physical pain she had been holding in. The pediatrician listened.

He looked at me and said, "I could order every test but I truly believe Rachel is suffering from depression." As soon as he said those words, I looked over at Rachel to see her head slowly nodding up and down as tears were silently running down her face. It was at that moment that I realized the impact the brace was having on her life.

Rachel: It's hard to explain how everything I was feeling was not the real me. The girl who was once so outgoing and happy was quickly disappearing. The colors began to fade away as I felt myself falling into this dark hole. Sleep became my great escape. I felt that if I were sleeping, it would be fewer hours awake in the brace.

Mom: I brought Rachel back to our orthopedist to share my concerns and asked her to look at the brace. After she examined the brace, she could see the areas that were causing Rachel's pain and bruises. She suggested bringing the brace back to the orthotist for adjustments.

We went back to this orthotist three more times and, unfortunately, the only thing that seemed to change was that the owner of the company became involved. I'm not sure why, as he made no difference.

Rachel: With each visit back to the orthotist, nothing ever changed. The orthotist was always cold and insensitive and I hated his condescending tone when he spoke to me; he only made me cry more.

Mom: "This cannot be a normal reaction when being fitted for a brace," I said to the orthotist.

He didn't respond. Was he ignoring me?

Seeing Rachel continue to cry made me even more upset.

"Stop, and just take the brace off of her," I finally said in a voice that even surprised me.

I once again insisted that something was wrong.

The last comment he made was, "She'll be fine. This is still an adjustment period she is going through." By now Rachel was hysterical, and we left.

Rachel: I had no choice but to continue to wear my suit of armor under my clothes. School was almost over and I was excited that I didn't have to deal with the dressing issue much longer. The only other activities that made me somewhat happy were my dance classes; there I was able to be brace-free for the hour. Unfortunately, as my back pain increased, dancing was becoming less enjoyable. After nine years of dance, I finally just gave it up.

I think one of the worst experiences I had with my back brace was a trip to the emergency room. Sharp pains shooting down my right leg and abdomen were so intense I wasn't even able to walk upstairs.

Mom: On the initial emergency room exams, Rachel was symptomatic for an inflamed appendix. As each emergency doctor gently pressed down on the lower right side of her abdomen, she jumped with pain. One of the attending physicians noticed Rachel's deep red marks toward the lower right side of her abdomen where her pain was located. He asked Rachel to show him how she wears the brace.

Rachel: Initially, I had no idea why the emergency room doctors were asking to see my back brace or have me put it on for them. Once on, I immediately flinched with pain as the bottom of the brace dug into my right lower abdomen. They observed the bruises and how it lined up right next to where my brace was digging into me and causing pain. A light bulb went on for one specific doctor when he realized my appendix was literally bruised by my back brace.

Mom: Having the emergency room doctor conclude that her brace was bruising her appendix made me angrier than any words I could ever express. Rachel was instructed to stop wearing the brace until changes were made to the brace and the inflammation subsided. As Rachel proceeded to get changed, I couldn't help but become furious. We trusted the "experts" to help our daughter, but it was apparent now that they didn't know what they were doing. The next day my husband returned their useless piece of plastic.

Rachel: I was out of the brace for several weeks until my abdomen healed. When I was finally able to resume bracing, I was happy that my parents found a more professional office to work with. My new orthotist, Steve Mullins, was kind and patient. He explained that bracing is never comfortable, but what he promised to do was make it as tolerable as possible. This experience was nothing like what I went through four months earlier. It was like we were working together. I told him where it hurt, and wherever he could, he made adjustments. I left there much happier than I ever expected. I was wearing the brace and not crying. I actually felt confident for the first time that I might be able to do this.

Mom: Watching Rachel being refitted for a new brace with no tears was amazing. The difference in her care was like night and day. When the new brace was completed, she said it was tight, but she could still breathe. Within a few days, Rachel was able to meet her required sixteen hours of bracing a day. As an extra bonus, when she was X-rayed again in her new brace, her curve decreased to 18°! This was a remarkable improvement from the previous brace, where the orthotist was only able to decrease her curve to 25°. And to think all of this was accomplished without any tears.

THEY DON'T UNDERSTAND

Rachel: Even though my bracing problems disappeared, my back pain never went away. My follow-up appointments were supposed to be every six months, but since I was still in so much back pain, I sometimes had to go back two months earlier.

Going to the doctor's was like listening to a broken record. I'd tell them I'm in pain and they'd basically say, "No you're not." I guess they really don't believe us when we tell them our backs or our hips hurt because the standard response seems to be, "There's no pain with scoliosis."

Instead, they turn it around and ask psychological questions: "How's everything going at home?" "Are you having problems with any friends?" "How are your grades?" "Do you struggle in any subjects?"

Like an obedient patient, I answered everything appropriately, but felt like this was the doctor's way of blaming my pain on something other than the scoliosis. What always confused me was why would I lie to the very people who were supposed to be helping me? It felt like my doctors didn't believe that my pain was real. Didn't they know how horrible that made me feel?

Mom: If Rachel wasn't complaining of so much back pain, I would have never looked at her back and seen how significant her scoliosis had progressed. Doesn't that tell you something? No one was ever able to answer this question.

Rachel: Needless to say, nothing ever came from these earlier visits. At times, I think my doctor actually felt bad that she couldn't explain why my back hurt so much.

Mom: Our orthopedist recommended that Rachel begin two or three days of physical therapy each week to strengthen muscles that were being weakened from bracing. She also wanted Rachel to be treated once a week by a particular therapist who would concentrate on muscle strengthening for children with scoliosis.

EVERYTHING HAPPENS FOR A REASON

Rachel: On the very first appointment with the physical therapist, she pointed out the parts of my body that were being weakened from the scoliosis. I have to admit, I was surprised how hard it was to do the simplest exercises. Since I was still suffering with pain primarily located in my mid and upper back, the therapist tried to work the problem area out with an aggressive massage.

Mom: Once again, Rachel did not seem to benefit from this particular therapist's method for relieving her pain. As nice as she was, Rachel was still in pain. I needed to find another alternative for treatment.

Rachel: I couldn't move; her hands were pressing very hard on certain areas of my back. I later learned that she was trying to release one of the many trigger points (muscle spasms) that I had all over my upper back. I knew after that session I was through with people trying to help me with my pain—at least for a while.

Mom: Ironically, it was at the end of this session when the therapist mentioned that there was another girl in the waiting area who also had scoliosis, and was starting a support group for kids. "Would you be interested in meeting her?"

Rachel: Up to this point, I never met anyone else with scoliosis. She handed me a flyer and told me about a support group she wanted to begin, and asked if I would be interested in going. I eagerly said "yes" and in turn I gave her my telephone number.

Rachel: People often tell me I'm an old soul because I tend to spend more time reflecting on why things have happened to me. Maybe it's true, but this trait has allowed me to realize certain things that others might have overlooked. For example, if I never went to this therapist, I would have never met Leah Stoltz, a young girl who would later become an important part of my life.

Mom: When I first met Leah, I was immediately impressed with how well she spoke. For being only thirteen, she was very mature. I was quickly drawn to her warm smile and courageous outlook regarding her condition. Already braced two years, for twenty-two hours a day, I listened in awe as she handed us a flyer announcing the start of her own support group for kids with scoliosis. It was her intention to share whatever she learned and then talk openly about the everyday challenges of bracing. Impressed with her positive attitude, I left optimistic that this group might be exactly what Rachel needed.

Several days later, Leah's mom, Robin, called. We talked for a while and I felt an instant connection with her. Now more than ever, I was truly getting excited about this support group. Before we ended our conversation, we mutually chose the date and the place of the first meeting. On Sunday, August 6, 2006, Rachel and I, along with two other moms and their daughters, arrived at their home.

I'M NOT ALONE

Rachel: Before the summer ended, I attended my first support group meeting at Leah's home. Scared at first, my nerves quickly disappeared as Leah began to talk to us about issues that affected her most when she was first braced, like clothing.

"Has this ever happened to you?" Leah asked as she held up a DKNY shirt. "You have your favorite shirt on over your brace and there are holes."

I remembered nodding my head and thinking to myself, "I'm not alone." Someone was verbally expressing the frustrations of wearing something you really like, maybe only once, and then having it ruined by something you hated … your brace.

As Leah continued to talk, she explained the importance of layering. She gave us tips on how to layer our clothes so the straps on our braces wouldn't be seen. I soon nicknamed her the "Queen of Layering." Leah's valuable tips on layering the clothes with a tank top on underneath to cover the bulkiness helped prevent the outer shirt from getting damaged. Leah also knew something about sleeping more comfortably at night. She suggested putting a pillow under our legs to balance the unevenness the brace put us in while lying down.

"Doing this little trick," Leah said, "will help you sleep more comfortably at night."

By the end of our first meeting I was blown away with everything I had just learned. On the way home, I went clothes shopping with my mom and actually had fun. That evening when I had to go to bed, I slept great. Do you want to know why? Because I slept with a pillow under my legs! Needless to say, I was very anxious to return the following month to learn more of Leah's "scoliosis survival skills."

Mom: As the girls walked off to talk privately about their issues, the moms began to bond about doctors, back braces, and the overwhelming frustrations of whether or not we were making the right decisions for our girls. By the end of our first meeting, both Rachel and I left their home smiling and feeling like a weight was just lifted from our shoulders.

Who would have ever thought that talking to strangers would have been so effective?

Rachel: Somehow each month, Leah knew what we needed to talk about. One month we might discuss our innermost feelings of wearing the brace, how and why we felt the brace changed us, the anxieties we had right before our next doctor's appointment, or the fears someone might be going through anticipating having corrective surgery. Other times we'd talk about the different obstacles we faced being teenage girls, like problems in school or the dreaded girl drama. One of the things that made me so proud to be part of this group was that there were no cliques, no popular girls, and no mean girls, just girls with scoliosis whose goal was to help each other.

Leah, being the oldest, was a great role model; she always knew what to say. I remember once telling her, and the group, that I was having problems with some girls in school. Her genuine concern for my situation meant so much to me. It wasn't so much what she said, (though it did help) but how she reacted and listened. No matter the topic of conversation, the bottom line was that we supported each other and developed our very own "scoli-family."

The bond we all made is hard to explain, but we knew we wanted to continue to reach out and help others. Eventually, we decided to name our support group, "Curvy Girls."

Who would have imagined a random meeting in a physical therapist's office would have led to this?

Mom: As the first year passed, Rachel continued to be closely monitored. At each follow-up appointment, we would learn if her curve progressed, if her Risser score went up, and if she grew any taller. Taking new X-rays every four months was something I hated putting Rachel through, but we had no choice. During this time, as Rachel grew, her curve basically remained the same. It would go up a couple of degrees and then back down. I attributed this success to Rachel's strict discipline on complying with her bracing. Never did I see her trying to cheat or even loosen her straps during those years.

Rachel: When I finally got my period, I was so excited. Most girls probably wouldn't have cared as much, but for a girl with scoliosis, getting your period means that an end to bracing is now in sight. The countdown had finally begun for me; I knew in two years my spine will have stopped growing and I will be brace-free. However, it was during this time that a few of the girls in our support group, who were braced longer than me, found out they needed surgery. This was a difficult time for me as I watched these girls, who I now considered my friends, prepare for surgery. I couldn't help but begin to wonder, "Am I wearing my brace for no reason? Will I end up having surgery just like them?"

Mom: I was surprised to hear Rachel question whether or not bracing was really worth it. I felt like I needed to discuss this further with her, fearing that she might begin to give up. I explained to Rachel that if these girls never wore their brace, their curves would have probably progressed to even a higher degree. Plus, the sad reality is that some kids might progress to the point of surgery regardless of how much they braced. No one knows for sure. All I do know is that giving up the brace is not the smartest decision, especially when we know the brace is working for you. Rachel later learned that some of the girls admitted they stopped wearing their brace consistently. They encouraged the other girls not to make the same mistake. On a positive note, within eight months of her first period, Rachel's pelvic growth plate (Risser) went from a 1 to a 4-5, which meant her growing was really coming to an end. I was so excited to share this great news with family and friends who were our anchors during this time.

REGAINING CONTROL

Rachel: By the end of the sixth grade, I was having a hard time bracing every day in school. On top of it being difficult to wear, I was dealing with insensitive teachers. Sitting or standing for long periods was very uncomfortable, and while not often, sometimes I needed to walk around or go to the nurse just to take a little break from the brace. I actually had a teacher make fun of me when I asked to go to the nurse twice in one week.

Not only was I embarrassed by his rude comments, now I was more determined than ever to find another solution for not bracing during school hours. When I shared what happened in school with my mom, she immediately spoke to the teacher about how inappropriately he spoke to me. The next day in school he took me aside and apologized. Even though he said he was sorry, this experience left me more uncomfortable and fearful to wear my brace to school.

It was at this time my mom agreed to change my bracing hours. I think she finally began to understand what I was going through on a daily basis. I would now wear my brace from 3 p.m. to 7 a.m., which made it easier to deal with the restrictions at home rather than in school. Teachers and classmates never fully understood how hard it was to wear this turtle shell corset under my clothes.

A simple thing like dropping your pen, paper, or book, which would take anyone only a second to retrieve, is a project for someone strapped in this medieval harness offering no flexibility.

Not wearing the brace to school was the best decision I think we ever made. I actually felt happier. I never had to be reminded to put the brace on or to be checked to see if it was put on tight enough. Would you believe that I actually didn't mind wearing the brace anymore? It was true. I actually felt better in the brace than I did out of it. It's amazing how much easier bracing became once I took back some control in my life.

Mom: Sadly, Rachel's back pain continued, and though I tried everything from physical therapy to chiropractic treatments, the only thing that actually gave her any relief was massage therapy. While continuing our monthly support group meetings, I soon learned there were many other girls who also suffered with back pain. It will always confuse me as to why doctors insist there is no pain associated with this scoliosis.

SEPTEMBER 15TH

Rachel: It seemed like the typical routine appointment. Each visit started out the same, X-rays and then waiting. This time however, I was feeling a little more nervous than usual about the X-ray results because I had a secret that I had kept to myself.

"Mom, I'm afraid I might have screwed everything up. I've slacked off an hour or two several times over the last few weeks, and now I'm worried that my curve might have gotten worse!" I quickly blurted out.

Jokingly, my mom remarked, "What is this, confession time? Relax. You've been so good. A couple of hours shouldn't have made that much of a difference." Having my mom say that did help, but I wasn't stupid. The X-ray results are the only thing I could go by.

Nervously waiting in the exam room, the physician assistant quickly opened the door and announced, "You're brace-free! Go ahead, get dressed. I'll give you a moment, and then we'll talk," as she gently closed the door.

Completely stunned by the words that just came out of her mouth, I turned to look at my mom as she rushed over to hug me and we both began to cry.

"It's over, Rachel. You did it," my mom whispered in my ear as the tears began to fall. When the physician's assistant returned, she opened the door and saw us crying.

"What's with the crying? This is happy news!"

Still crying, I managed to say, "You don't understand how hard this was for me, and now you're telling me it's over. It doesn't seem real."

She smiled and said, "You can put a girl in a brace and she'll cry, take her out and she'll still cry!"

Mom: Rachel beat the odds. From the first day we were told she needed to be braced, we were forewarned that there was a strong likelihood she would end up needing corrective spine surgery. Unfortunately, my daughter had everything going against her. She was an eleven-year-old with a zero Risser, and a 35° curve which meant she still had a lot of growing to do. Our only option was to brace and monitor her growth. Needless to say, this process of "wait-and-see" left us all very anxious and frightened. And yet we did it. No, I stand corrected, Rachel did it; she beat the odds!

Today, when I reflect on everything she has gone through over these past few years, I'm overwhelmed with pride. I cannot adequately express how amazed I am by the strength that she found within herself at such a young age.

A few years ago, Rachel let me read a journal entry she had written in the sixth grade. The theme was, "If you had a chance to change one thing about yourself, what would it be?" Though most children her age would have written, "not to have scoliosis" or "not to have to wear a back brace," Rachel chose "nothing" and explained why. She wrote, "We all have obstacles in our life we're meant to overcome, and dealing with scoliosis must be mine." Rachel concluded that if she wished her scoliosis away, it would have been like wishing a part of her didn't exist.

I WOULDN'T CHANGE A THING

Rachel: I couldn't believe that my journey had ended. No more holes in my shirt, no more awkward sleeping positions, no more back brace! I walked out of that office happier than I could have ever thought imaginable. Once in the car, my mom and I joked that I just received a belated birthday gift, since my birthday had just passed on September 1st. Before we left the parking lot, my mom began calling everyone in the family to tell them that I was brace-free. I, unfortunately, couldn't stop crying, but continued to repeat the words, "I'm free; I'm really free." This new reality took a while for me to process.

There's no doubt in my mind that I could not have accomplished two-and-a-half years of bracing without the support from my family and the Curvy Girls. Having scoliosis made me grow up a lot faster than other kids my age. Coping with the drama in middle school and high school is difficult enough, but when you add scoliosis and bracing into the mix, it's overwhelming.

If you are reading my story right now, and you're depressed and suffering with your brace, don't start hating life because of this condition. Please learn from the mistakes we made through my bracing. Remember, bracing isn't comfortable, but it is bearable. If you're in pain with your brace, speak up. Allow our personal journeys to give you the confidence that we once lacked.

The diagnosis of scoliosis first changed me for the worst, and then inspired me to become a better person. If given the opportunity to change my past, I wouldn't change a thing.

After Rachel was discharged from bracing, her scoliosis journey did not come to an end as we anticipated. To find out how her story continued, read *Taking "Back" Control*.

WHERE RACHEL IS TODAY

After high school she attended college at the University of Rhode Island. In 2017, Rachel earned her Bachelor of Science where her academics focused on health promotion and disease prevention. After graduating, she went on to expand her areas of interest in public health by working at Memorial Sloan Kettering Cancer Center for three years. The role she has had at this institution greatly impacted her, as she now attends Brown University for a Master of Public Health, concentrating in epidemiology. As an epidemiologist, her goal is to conduct research and create interventional programs centered on cancer prevention through nutritional and environmental health sectors.

While she is transitioning in her career, Curvy Girls remains a significant part of her life. Since 2012, Rachel has co-led and co-created Curvy Girls' international biennial conventions. In 2014, she became the Vice President of the organization and also volunteered her time as Mentor to train other leaders around the globe.

Mimi

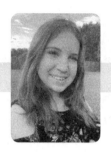

Meet Mimi from Florida

Age: 14

Braced at age 6

Magec Rods at age 10 – Spinal Fusion at age 13

Mimi enjoys reading, acting and hanging out with her friends.

Mimi has shared that Curvy Girls changed her life and put her on the path of helping others.

Mimi's story speaks to strength and resilience. When you look up the word "resilient" in the English dictionary, it says "able to withstand or recover quickly from difficult conditions." This is exactly what Mimi has done, and continues to do in spite of the challenges that have come her way.

Mimi's Message: It's so important to find other girls who can understand what you are going through.

Mimi Macklin and her mother, Julie Macklin

Finding the Magic

Mimi: For more than half of my life, I have been aware that I have scoliosis. I was told that I had juvenile idiopathic scoliosis when I was six years old. Being diagnosed so young sometimes makes it hard to tell the difference between my actual memories and what I was told. The diagnosis didn't mean anything to me at the time, but it certainly meant something to my mom, who also has scoliosis. The initial red flag occurred during a back-to-school, well visit appointment.

Mom: What had begun as a normal "check-up" to the pediatrician with my perfectly healthy six-year-old suddenly took an unexpected turn. We entered the office visit without a care in the world and within five minutes I was in shock and disbelief.

As the doctor handed me the referral for a spinal X-ray, memories of my own childhood experience came flooding back as I was diagnosed with scoliosis at ten years old. My doctor's explanation was that I grew "too fast."

But how was this happening to my petite little girl? She was just six years old. She's too young. I didn't have more than a few minutes to think about what I had just heard when she was sent out for X-rays.

The X-rays confirmed Mimi had juvenile idiopathic scoliosis with a fairly advanced curve of 35°. The unmistakable image of the prominent S curve in that first X-ray remains etched in my mind. I didn't understand how this could have happened to my first-born at such a young age.

Mimi: My first true memory was the day my mom took me to be fitted for my scoliosis brace. Confused as to why I needed to have this, my mom explained my back was like hers and that she also wore a brace when she was a child. The brace would help my spine stay straight as I grew, like it did for her and that made sense to me.

Mom: With more questions than answers from the doctor at this point, I did my best to explain to Mimi that although she couldn't feel anything, her back was not growing correctly. It was heartbreaking because

I knew from my own experiences with scoliosis and wearing a brace that this was not going to be easy. I also realized that such a severe curve at this young age would be difficult to fix.

Mimi: Getting fitted for a brace did not bother me. I was actually very excited when they told me I could design my brace the way I wanted it to look. This was harder than I thought because there were so many great patterns to choose from. I did manage to leave the orthotist's office that day with a smile on my face knowing my new Boston Brace was going to have purple and pink butterflies.

A few weeks later, we returned to pick up my brace. It was beautiful! I also didn't think it was a big deal, so when I came home, I showed all my friends. They were all very supportive and thought it was kind of cool looking. It did take a little while to get used to but once I did, I was able to do everything that most six-year-olds do—ride bikes, play with friends, and go swimming.

Mom: At first, Mimi took things in stride. The brace could be removed for bathing and swimming. Plus, it was white with purple and pink butterflies so she thought it was kind of cool. While initially uncomfortable, she did adapt. And after some early protests, she wore it without too much complaining. We thought everything was going well until doctors told us the brace was not effective at preventing her curve from progressing. We were devastated! After eighteen months of wearing her brace, her curve increased to nearly 45°.

CASTING

Mimi: When we found out that my curves progressed, my doctor recommended a body cast. This was the same kind of cast you'd wear if you broke your arm or leg—only much larger. He explained that putting a cast on my back would keep my spine straighter for a longer period of time—which would give me better results.

Mom: Mimi would have to be put under general anesthesia to have the cast applied. The procedure would be done on a special "rack" that would hold her spine in place as the casting material was wrapped around her body. The cast needed to stay on for six weeks and not get wet. The cast would then be removed for 24 hours with a new one applied and worn for another 6 weeks.

Mimi: Being only seven years old and hearing what was involved left me feeling pretty scared. To make matters worse, I couldn't take the cast off for six weeks. Realizing what I had to go through just made me cry. My parents did their best to help me feel better but I was still scared and didn't want to do this.

Waking up with the body cast on was a horrible nightmare. My first memory was feeling like I couldn't breathe. At that same moment I also realized that I couldn't move—the cast was extremely tight. Not feeling like I could breathe or move, I was scared and immediately began to cry. Unfortunately, the more upset I became, the worse I felt. That day was by far the hardest I had gone through in my life. My mom tried to keep me calm by reassuring me that this was not going to be forever. But at that moment, it truly felt like it.

Mom: Mimi did not like the cast at all and started asking questions about why this had happened to her and when it would be over. I struggled to find the right words to comfort her. I turned to my faith and explained that God had given her a special challenge and someday this would make her a stronger person. Without a doubt, this was a trying part of her journey.

Mimi: Over the next few days, I was grateful as the cast started to loosen up. I still wasn't happy wearing it but at least I felt more comfortable breathing. Going back to school I was greeted by my friends and classmates who were always very kind and supportive. Even my teacher surprised me and allowed everyone to sign my body cast at the playground. I really appreciated how concerned and helpful all the students were —from helping me pick up something that I dropped to carrying my backpack.

Mom: Going six weeks at a time without a bath was hard for my water-loving girl who was now eight. Adding to these difficult months I was also pregnant at the time with her sister, so bathing Mimi was not an easy task. I had to wash her hair in the kitchen sink and then sponge bathe her on the side of the tub. As hard as it was, I didn't care as long as it enabled that cast to do its job.

Mimi: During those months in the body cast, I tried my best to be like everyone else but that wasn't easy. Life in a cast had a lot of limitations and there were many things that my friends could do that were off limits for me. Most days I felt frustrated, angry and sad. What made some days worse than others was seeing my friends in the pool or playing in their sprinklers. All I could do was watch because I was not allowed to get the cast wet. And if the cast couldn't get wet, that also meant no baths or showers.

Finally, after 6 weeks of waiting, the first cast was removed! I now had 24 hours to celebrate before the second cast was put on. I took full advantage of enjoying every second being out of that cast. To celebrate, I took three baths that day just because I could. I did everything I hadn't been able to do—ride my bike, run, and swim in the pool. I felt free!

Getting the second cast put on was a little easier since I knew what to expect. I'd have to live with it for six weeks. Then it would come off and I'd be free again—or at least that's what I thought. But when the doctor sent me for X-rays to see how I was doing, there was a problem. The cast hadn't been as effective as the doctor had hoped. That's when everything changed.

Mom: We had moments of optimism when we would see how nearly perfect her spine looked while in the cast, but our hopes were completely shattered when the cast came off and her spine quickly progressed to more than 50°. Unfortunately, these difficult times were only a preview of what was to come.

The surgeon tried two more rounds of casting, but it was never effective. With her curve approaching 70° post-cast, the doctor gave us the news that Mimi would require a major surgery to implant growing rods. The extendable rods would be fixed under the skin to her top and bottom vertebrae to straighten the curve. This meant that every six months, for the next five-to-six years, Mimi would need minor surgeries to extend the rods which would allow her spine to grow to its natural height. Then around age 14-16, her spine would need to be permanently fused. With Mimi now nine years old, she would require 20 more surgeries to get to a final solution. Nothing about this sounded good, so before making a decision we sought out a second opinion with one of the most renowned pediatric orthopedic surgeons in the country.

FACING SURGERY

Mimi: With bracing no longer an option, my parents took me to see a new doctor. He told us about a brand new surgical procedure using something called MAGEC growing rods. This would involve fewer surgeries but I would have to return every couple of months to lengthen my spine with a magnet held against my back. This sounded kind of exciting to me. Plus, I would be one of the first patients to try this new device. My parents seemed to think this was the best option for me, so surgery was scheduled.

Mom: Without hesitation, we drove six hours to Miami Children's Hospital. The initial evaluation confirmed the need for more aggressive treatment but offered a bit of hope in the possibility of a new type of growing rod. The initial procedure was the same, but these new "MAGEC Rods" could be lengthened in a brief office visit every three or four months. A special motor driver would actuate magnets built into the rods causing them to rotate and extend. This would eliminate the need for the invasive biannual surgical adjustments. Unfortunately, there was a problem. The new treatment was not yet approved by the FDA—and that process could take another full year or more. As a solution, the surgeon suggested keeping Mimi in casts as long as possible, hoping when the device was approved, we would then be able to use the MAGEC Rods.

Much to our surprise, a week after scheduling another cast application, we got a call that the MAGEC rods had been FDA-approved. Mimi would actually be one of the first patients in the country to receive the new rods, which would hopefully get her through until the final fusion. This meant that our daughter would only need one single surgery, not twenty. Finally, we had a break!

Although apprehensive about committing to this major procedure, we felt it was the best treatment option and agreed to proceed. A few weeks later, we packed up everything (including Mimi's 11-month-old-sister) and headed south.

Mimi: Since this was my first major operation, I was very nervous. I didn't know what to expect and I didn't have anyone to talk to because no one else had this surgery yet. When the surgery was over there was definitely pain, but I was told that was normal. Every day I got a little stronger and by the end of the week, we were heading home.

Two months later, we returned to the hospital where the doctor used the special magnet to extend the rods to lengthen my spine. We would repeat those visits every month for the next three years. The only complaint I had after they lengthened my spine was the sensation of pins and needles on my back, but these symptoms went away in a few days.

Everything was going as planned until I had another problem. I found out I needed to have a second surgery. One of the surgical screws came loose, which required them to replace the growing rods.

Mom: Mimi went into the surgery with a positive attitude; however, the recovery pain from replacing the growing rods was more than any of us expected. She became very upset and moody, at times completely inconsolable. Although she had amazing support from friends and family, she was quick-tempered with them, as well as with her father and me. My super positive and strong girl was now a completely different person.

FINDING CURVY GIRLS

Mimi: Going through two major surgeries in a short amount of time took a huge toll on me both physically and emotionally. While recovering in the hospital after the second surgery, my mom noticed I wasn't doing that well emotionally. I was ten years old; I had been through a lot and wasn't as happy as I once was. I also didn't know how to make myself feel better. That's when I found out that my mom was searching on the internet for some kind of support for me.

Mom: Looking for answers, I began searching on the internet for scoliosis support groups and found Curvy Girls. Online, we read the stories about other girls with scoliosis. Mimi became encouraged when she discovered she wasn't alone. She immediately lit up and wanted to be involved.

Mimi: I was so excited when my mom showed me the Curvy Girls' website. We wanted to attend a meeting but it wasn't possible because the nearest group was five hours away. That's when my mom asked me if I'd like to start my own chapter. I immediately perked up again and said yes. The next thing we did was write to the Foundation to ask if I could be the leader in this part of Florida.

When I got the news that I was going to become the leader of a Curvy Girls' chapter, I was delighted! At age 10, I became the head of the North

Central Florida chapter (with a little help from my mom). I couldn't wait to help people just like me! Having the support from other girls who are going through the same thing is so important to this journey.

Mom: Once we received approval, I saw an immediate change in Mimi. Even though she was still in a lot of pain, her attitude completely shifted. She felt more confident and happier knowing that she could now help other girls like herself.

Mimi: Shortly after becoming a leader, we found out there was a Curvy Girls' convention scheduled and I couldn't wait to go. I quickly learned that meeting other girls that have scoliosis can help decrease anxiety just by talking to each other.

Mom: Being a part of Curvy Girls gave us the opportunity to attend their biennial international conferences. As a new leader Mimi also attended the leadership training. Here we not only learned more about scoliosis, but Mimi got to meet so many girls like herself. On that first day she became instant friends with several of her peers. Now armed with some common connections and a greater understanding of scoliosis, the trip was a game changer for our entire family. Connecting her experience to a larger group was empowering and completely changed her outlook for the better.

Mimi: Walking into the hotel where the convention was being held and seeing so many girls wearing Curvy Girls' tee shirts and wearing their scoliosis braces made me feel like I belonged. Looking at everyone in the hotel lobby that day left me kind of speechless. I was also beyond happy because for the first time ever, I felt like I wasn't alone anymore. Though a lot of us were meeting each other for the first time, it didn't take long before we bonded and became best of friends. After one workshop with Leah and Rachel, I couldn't believe how much we all had in common. That's when I realized how important it is to have friends that can understand firsthand what you are going through. By the third and final day of the convention, I had already become close friends with two of the girls that I met. What an unexpected gift to get from attending my very first Curvy Girls' convention!

THE MAGIC OF SUPPORT

Mom: Two years later we were told that Mimi was not getting any more length out of one of her rods because one of the screws had come loose. This would require yet another surgery to fix the rods. This news did not go over very well with Mimi. Sharing her story with her Curvy Girls' friends, and receiving their encouragement and support, she was able to have a positive attitude the whole time. Although it was still difficult, she was emotionally solid this time. Even the friends that visited after the first surgery noticed the difference.

Mimi: Having the support of Curvy Girls around the world made a big difference then, and even three years later when I learned the MAGEC RODS stopped lengthening. This was something I knew would eventually happen, except it was four years sooner than we had anticipated. As scared as I was to have the final surgery—spinal fusion, I knew it was time. By now I was in terrible back pain every day and unable to do any kind of physical activity.

Mom: After one brace, two casts and two growing rod surgeries in seven years, the time had come when she needed to have the spinal fusion surgery at 13 years old. The rods had reached their maximum length and Mimi was now in chronic pain. Over-the-counter pain medication and physical therapy were not helping. We had to make the call that it was time to take the rods out and fuse her spine. Realistically, the devices had served their purpose. It was always meant to be a temporary fix to keep her curve from getting worse in order to get the best possible correction when it was time to fuse.

Mimi: During the weeks leading up to the surgery, it helped knowing I could share my fears and questions with any of the girls that I met at the convention or the Curvy Girls' discussion forum. I felt very lucky to have so many people trying to help me, including my school friends. The weekend before my surgery, my friends gathered at my house for an ice cream social to help me get my mind off the big day.

Mom: Once again Mimi went into this surgery with a positive attitude. She did have times when her emotions were high and she had anxiety. But to be honest, who wouldn't be nervous or on edge? These were definitely challenging days.

Mimi: As prepared as I thought I was, I was still very nervous the morning of the surgery. I went into the operating room pretty scared but also anxious to just have it over. Waking up after the surgery the pain was pretty bad. I can honestly say that recovering from this surgery was by far the hardest of all the procedures I'd been through. When friends came to visit me in the hospital, I tried my best to seem okay when I really wasn't.

Mom: Since this was not Mimi's first surgery, she knew the sooner she got up out of bed and walked the sooner she would recover. The day after her surgery she was walking a lap around the nurses' station with the physical therapist. Any chance she had, she was sitting in a chair.

Mimi: I forced myself to push through the pain every day because I knew from my other surgeries that the sooner you stand up and walk, the faster you heal. So regardless of how bad I felt the day after surgery, I got up and did a lap around the PICU with the physical therapist. I focused on getting up, walking, sitting in the chair as much as I could without overdoing it.

My first three or four months had more bad days then good, but eventually everything did improve and life picked up right where I left off.

Mom: Once again, Mimi had lots of visitors to distract her as she recovered at home. I cannot stress how important it is to have people come and play games or just watch a TV show with your daughter in between resting. It gives them something to look forward to and a diversion from the pain.

Two weeks after surgery, she was ready to go back to school part-time. I emailed all her teachers a few days before and asked if she could bring a pillow, leave class a few minutes before the bell rang, and have a helper who could wheel her backpack. Thankfully, everyone was onboard and very accommodating. I even got permission to have her eat outside with a friend to avoid getting bumped and jostled in the busy cafeteria. For the first week-and-a-half she attended her first four classes of the day and then I would pick her up early.

Three months after spinal fusion, Mimi was back on stage rehearsing for a play at our local state theater. A month later, she was performing five shows a week for an entire month. Six months later you would never know she even had surgery—other than she is a few inches taller. For the first time in eight years, we only have to see her doctor once a year instead of every two or three months.

PERSONAL TIPS

Mimi: After having three surgeries, I can tell you the best thing to do when you get home is to schedule people to come over for short visits. This helps to get your mind off any pain you are still feeling. I also believe you should keep a positive attitude during the healing process. Before my surgery, people sent me colored cards that had inspirational quotes on them; those cards helped keep me motivated during my recovery.

If you are having surgery while school is in session, it is key to communicate with your teachers and administration in advance. A few weeks before my surgery date, I asked my teachers for the work I was going to miss so I wouldn't fall behind. For my return back to school, special arrangements were made to avoid being in the hallways with everyone at the same time. Believe it or not, I went back to school two weeks after my surgery, but only for a few classes. I slowly worked my way up to a full day.

FINAL THOUGHTS

Mom: While our story is coming to an end, your journey might just be beginning. Allow me to share a few things we have learned over the past eight years.

Though it's wonderful to have family support, it's important to have support from families who are going through what you are. That is what Curvy Girls has given to us and can offer you. Don't be afraid or uncomfortable to ask for second or third opinions. Do your research and get a good understanding on which brace might work best for your child's curve. Just like what we are told—no two curves are alike, and neither are any two braces. If your daughter is in pain, find a certified physical therapist trained in scoliosis-specific exercises.

If surgery becomes an option, ask for input from parents whose child has already had fusion. How was their experience? Learn more about non-fusion surgeries and see if your child is a candidate.

We often hear people say that it's the hard times that make us who we are. Well, that is apparently true because today if Mimi sees other kids in need, she is always eager to help. Whether it's sitting with a child with special needs at lunch because no one else does, or playing with a ten-year-old girl staying with her grandparents next door while awaiting cancer treatment, she is the first to jump in and give support. For someone so young, she knows the importance of helping others not feel alone. The journey certainly has not been easy, but it has truly shaped who Mimi is today—a very loving, compassionate girl who handles life with the grace of a young adult, while continuing to use her scoliosis experiences to help others.

LIFE AFTER SCOLIOSIS

Mimi: I'm not going to lie—having the physical treatment of scoliosis over is a great feeling!

When I started this journey, I knew I had a lot of love and support from my mom, dad and sister. But what I did not know is that I had another family made up of girls from all around the world through the Curvy Girls Scoliosis Foundation! The people I've met have inspired me to concentrate more fully on helping others deal with their own scoliosis journeys. One of the things I appreciate most about Curvy Girls is the tools and lessons I've learned that I can apply while helping someone, with or without scoliosis! It's amazing what kind of impact you can leave by offering someone a hand in friendship or an ear to listen.

> ### WHERE MIMI IS TODAY
> *Today, Mimi remains the Curvy Girls' chapter leader in her hometown. Her strength and determination to persevere through countless surgeries serves as her motivation to give back. Her goal is to carry on the Curvy Girls' domino effect of kindness by working with kids as either a youth leader or a teacher. Mimi is also active in community theatre and Girls Scouts of America.*

Alyssa

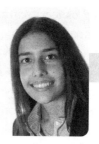

Meet Alyssa from England

Age: 16

Braced at age 12 with on-going scoliosis specific physiotherapy.

Alyssa enjoys sports, such as netball and tennis. Music is also a big part of her life; she plays both the clarinet and the piano. Alyssa particularly enjoys playing film scores. She dedicates her spare time to voluntary work at her local hospital and, of course, Curvy Girls!

Curvy Girls helped Alyssa realize that by embracing her insecurities, she can turn them into her strengths.

A scoliosis diagnosis led her to a downward spiral of endless secrets and feelings of isolation until she heard that her idol, Martha Hunt, also had scoliosis and was partnered with Curvy Girls. Over time, Alyssa's imperfect curves become a source of pride.

Alyssa's Message: Scoliosis shouldn't hold you back. With the right help and support you can pursue your dreams, ambitions and be yourself—your own kind of normal.

Alyssa Dunlop and her mother, Jusna Dunlop

My Kind of Normal

Alyssa

Some days and moments in life stand out so vividly you can't be sure they didn't happen yesterday. Or, you replay them so often you can't be sure they really happened. For me, the end of December was such a period. It was then that my mother discovered that I had scoliosis.

I was 12 years old and had been experiencing back pain for a while. However, each time I saw my general practitioner (GP), my pain was dismissed as growing pains, which was apparently normal for girls my age.

During these years, my favorite pastime was participating in all kinds of sports. I lived for playing netball, hockey, and tennis and took every single opportunity I could to play. I also loved hanging out with friends, going into town, buying new clothes—typical endeavors for a girl on the brink of her teenage years. Overall, you could say I was living my life to the fullest and just trying to fit in with everyone else—which made what happened next so much harder.

I was in the centre of Bath, a small quaint town in England, with my mum trying on clothes that I hoped to wear on Christmas day. Despite it being the 'most wonderful time of the year,' I remember feeling quite exhausted that day. I had been in a significant amount of back pain and just wanted to sit down. Nevertheless, I managed to find a blue jumpsuit that was perfect for the occasion and went into one of the changing rooms to try it on. I walked out, needing my mum to zip up the back for me when I heard her laugh. She said that I'd forgotten to take out the tissue paper in the back of the jumpsuit. But I was confused; there was no tissue paper.

The smile on her face dropped. She reached her hand out towards my spine and I heard her inhale as she touched it. My right shoulder blade was protruding so much she thought it couldn't have been my actual back. I could sense her worry as she traced my lopsided and uneven spine with the tips of her fingers. As much as she tried to hide it, I knew deep down that something was wrong. Despite this, I decided to push it to the side and not worry. I just wanted to enjoy the holidays and assumed that whatever it was, it was only temporary and I would recover as if it were the common cold.

A few days passed and I'd all but forgotten about the incident with my mother. That's why when my dad casually offered to take me out for breakfast before his physiotherapy appointment, I thought nothing of it and went to keep him company. I remember sitting through the session being relatively bored, waiting for it to be over. When we were finally ready to go, he suddenly turned to the physiotherapist and told him about what had happened that day in the changing room. Without hesitation, the physio asked to look at my back.

There was an uneasy silence in the room as he examined my spine. He then declared that I might have a condition called 'scoliosis.' I don't remember much else that day because the word meant nothing to me. Nevertheless, I politely listened to what the physiotherapist said. Because he was calm in explaining the condition, there was no reason for me not to be as well. He recommended that we look into a specialized type of physiotherapy for scoliosis in London. The physiotherapist assured me that this specific program could help to control my pain and condition. He explained that I'd have to learn a certain set of exercises and that I would probably have to miss school for two weeks. That didn't seem like such a bad tradeoff—I would be out of school for a couple of weeks, get a trip to London, and everything would go back to the way it had been before my mum saw my back in the changing room. At that point, it didn't sound like scoliosis was going to change my life at all.

THE DIAGNOSIS

The next few weeks flew by. My mum and I went to see my GP once again after the physiotherapist appointment and she confirmed that I did in fact have scoliosis. The doctor explained to my mum that scoliosis is a condition that prevents the spine from growing straight. My spine had a curve. The GP recommended that I see an orthopedic surgeon and have both an X-ray and an MRI scan done of my spine.

I can't fully explain why, but that hospital visit was more thrilling to me than anything else! I remember my first X-ray as if it were yesterday, and putting on the hospital gown for the first time and not knowing how to tie it up. Then, the loud whirring sound of the massive MRI machine as it created a three-dimensional image of my spine. I remember, too, the twisting feeling in my stomach when I looked at the results with my mum and the surgeon. I stared at the image with my eyes fixated on the notable kink in the top right of my spine. This wasn't what I had anticipated, but I put my trust in what the physiotherapist had told my dad and me. I convinced myself that it was going to be okay. I didn't stress; I didn't fret.

"You're going to need surgery," the surgeon stated bluntly. "You're going to lose almost all flexibility in your spine, so you won't be able to play sports. It has to be done because your current curvature is at 56°."

I stared blankly at him. Surgery? No one had mentioned that to me before. My heart began racing and my face grew hot as I struggled to hold back tears. I was angry, upset, and confused. The physiotherapist made it seem like this was no big deal but the surgeon made my diagnosis sound devastating. How could he just announce that to me, as if it meant nothing?

Suddenly scoliosis was no longer an excuse to go to London or a cool story I could tell my friends. This was serious. Everything around me became dizzy as I thought about the reality of my condition. No more sports; no more flexibility. How could that be? I had just learned how to do splits. How could it be that I might not be able to walk properly! I wouldn't let this happen; I just couldn't imagine that kind of future. Fortunately for me, my parents couldn't envision major surgery for me either and they resolved to look at alternative treatments.

There are moments like this in my life when I realize how lucky I am to have my parents. They didn't talk to me much about what was going to happen, but they assured me that there were other options we could explore—and that whatever happened, it would be for the best. My experience taught me a very valuable lesson:

Don't blindly follow someone's advice just because they are a "professional."

PHYSIO

Within a matter of days, my mum had looked into the option of specialized physiotherapy for scoliosis. With my approval, she booked me in for the two-week course in London. Making that one decision, and having that appointment planned, made me feel as if a large weight had been lifted off my chest. There was a downside though. Because I was still growing, I needed to have regular visits with an orthopedic surgeon to monitor the progress of my curvature. I agreed, provided I didn't have to visit the same one as before. To my luck, my mum had already found an alternative surgeon who saw other options than just surgery. Fast forward four years and I'm still visiting that same surgeon today, but only for periodic evaluations.

Once I understood the severity of my scoliosis, I was determined to successfully complete the physiotherapy course and stick to the exercise regimen. When the day came to start the two-week intensive course at the clinic in London, I remember being very nervous. At my first session, everyone was so welcoming that I would soon learn there was nothing to be worried about. I enjoyed those two weeks, and loved seeing the variety of people who live and thrive while having scoliosis. They made me feel a little less alone. I learned new exercises, improved my posture and was educated about my scoliosis and the nature of my curve. To make matters even better, at the end of the two weeks, my scoliosis had shown a massive improvement in rotation! I would need to spend 45 minutes every day doing exercises for my back and spine. I was relieved to know that this would enable me to live a normal life, and no one would ever have to know about my scoliosis.

But then my parents sat me down and told me those dreaded words that no 12-year-old girl could ever prepare herself to hear. I needed to wear a back brace. My face fell. What? How could they do this to me? Every pretense of being calm and collected about my condition had now completely disappeared. Suddenly surgery didn't seem so bad in the face of this devastating piece of news.

I didn't think matters could get any worse until they told me I'd have to wear the brace 23 hours per day. Every day? What about sports? What about school? As far as I was concerned, I couldn't wear a back brace—not at school, not anywhere. I shouted at my parents, cried at them— begging them not to ruin my life, but they kept insisting it was 'for the best.'

I pleaded that the physiotherapy was more than enough and I relentlessly argued against the redundancy of being strapped into a bulky plastic corset, but it was useless. In that moment, I felt helpless. Nothing I could say or do would change their minds. For the next month, I hopelessly savored every minute I had left of my "back brace-free life." I kept telling myself that the decision wasn't final, but each day passed and nothing changed; I was still getting the brace.

BRACE LIFE

The journey to Cardiff, where I would be fitted, was one of the worst days of my life. I contemplated jumping out of the car and making a run for it. No song was loud enough to drown out the fact that my world was ending. When we finally arrived I was still very angry, but the clinician there did his best to make this appointment as painless as possible. Fortunately, the fitting itself went relatively smoothly. Once I had had all my measurements taken it was only a matter of time until my next appointment was scheduled. Before I knew it, I was back in the treatment center awaiting the reveal of the notorious brace I had been so intensely dreading.

What I had thought to be a brace didn't come close to what I was given. Instead, it was rather a humongous, awkwardly-shaped object plonked before my eyes. That can't be right. I was not about to wear THAT. I repulsively examined its protruding bumps and curves and hastily decided that I hated it. Making it pink didn't disguise how disgustingly awful it was. I tried it on, hoping that it would at least feel comfortable, but no. It was cold and sticky and it scratched against my underarms. It dug into me in awkward places and I could barely move or bend—I felt practically immobile. I left the center that day more upset than I had ever been, struggling to hold back tears on the journey home. I eventually caved in that night and broke down in the confinement of my bedroom. Why me? Why do I have to be the one with scoliosis?

A few days passed and I began to get more comfortable with my brace, although it was starting to give me blisters where it dug in. As a result, I hadn't left the house in a while, but with school creeping closer, I had to complete a task that I had feared for a while: uniform shopping. Nearly every school in the United Kingdom requires a uniform for students, which meant I had to go out and buy new items in a much larger size to fit over my back brace. I prayed that I would be able to find the right items that could hide it, but no matter how hard I tried, you could still see the brace's bulky outline underneath my clothes. I stared at myself in the mirror with disgust and wept. I looked hulky and frumpy from every angle and I couldn't even imagine going into school dressed like this. But I did, and I despised it.

Attending school with a back brace is a universal challenge. I hadn't realized how many things I had long taken for granted, such as getting changed for sports or simply bending down to tie my shoes. Simple tasks that I had previously done with no thought were now mammoth, stress-inducing mountains to climb. I was fortunate to have a supportive school; they did everything they could to make life with a back brace more manageable for me. But as much as I needed the school officials' help, I didn't want it. I just wanted my scoliosis to go away. I wanted to be normal. Even with their help, every day for me was a struggle. To make matters worse, my friends at the time weren't that supportive. Instead of encouraging me to wear my back brace and use the facilities that the school had provided for me, they were equally as embarrassed as I was, almost as if I stood out—they would too. They refused to use the chairs with me during assembly, so I often found myself crouching on the floor with everyone else and getting laughed at by the girls behind me who found my brace protruding through my oversized school jumper amusing. I tried to ignore it, but their giggles were just a constant reminder of how different I was and how different I thought I'd always feel.

This led to me skipping school assemblies completely, as I couldn't handle the constant anxiety of being looked at. Sometimes it was more than just looking, as people would knock on my back and point. As much as I tried to be strong about it, all it did was make me weak. I was determined to carry on as if everything was normal. But in reality, I felt far from normal and every single day was a challenge.

This delicate relationship with my back brace continued for another two years as I tried to navigate my way through senior high school. Although the brace was becoming more comfortable to wear, and I no longer had blisters, I was still as insecure about it as I had always been. Very few people in my school knew that I had one, as I continued to go to extensive measures to conceal it. I grew my hair out so it would cover the top of my brace, yet still freaked out whenever someone walked closely behind me. And the minefield of school assemblies made me just as stressed and uncomfortable as they always had. I avoided every mirror I could so that I didn't upset myself, and I still refused to sit on my 'special chair' in science lessons. Really, nothing had changed except one thing: everyone else.

FRIENDSHIPS CHANGE

I was now 14 years old and surrounding myself with completely different people than those I was with when I first got diagnosed. In a way, that's understandable because friendships, like people, change over time. But I soon felt as if my new friends didn't like me the way they liked each other. When I compared myself to them, I identified the characteristic that singled me out from the rest of them—my scoliosis and back brace. They were all pretty and popular while I hated every part about myself, especially my scoliosis. They loved dressing up and taking pictures—things I didn't feel comfortable doing in a back brace. I could barely go to the supermarket without feeling self-conscious, let alone a party. Those girls would never understand what I was going through and, as time passed, I just felt more and more alone. It got to the point where I could barely wake up in the morning without reminding myself of my worthlessness. I had become a tearful, withdrawn, shell of a girl. Unfortunately, this new group of friends were quick to decide that I wasn't worth the trouble and moved on without me, pushing me further into a state of depression. I had lost my friends because of my scoliosis. I was no longer that easy-going social person I once was, which made me feel like I had lost a part of myself.

My family also noticed the changes in my attitude and tried to help—my sister even suggested counseling. But what could a therapist do to fix my spine? It seemed as if things would never change, until one day my sister discovered that the supermodel Martha Hunt also has scoliosis, and is a proud ambassador of an organization designed to support young girls suffering from the condition. The organization was called Curvy Girls. My sister convinced me to write to them, which helped me realize that I wasn't alone. There was hope.

NEW DIRECTION

After learning that Curvy Girls didn't have any chapters in England, I was even more determined to help start one. I knew that there must be other girls just like me who were experiencing the same challenges with scoliosis and needed help. Within months, I became the official Curvy Girls England chapter leader and I was off to my first Curvy Girls International Scoliosis Conference in New York with my mum! After what felt like forever, I was finally excited about something. If being part of the organization made me feel normal, then meeting over 300 girls with scoliosis from all around the world made me feel invincible.

There are no words to describe how amazing it was to be surrounded by girls just like me. We were all from different parts of the world, with different backstories and different treatment plans. But deep inside we shared many of the same fears and dreams.

We wanted to be accepted for who we were and not the medical condition that made us "different" from other girls.

Nobody at the conference let their condition define them, which helped me to see that I shouldn't try to hide this part of myself. I can honestly say that I walked away from that convention being the most confident I had been since my diagnosis.

My experience there had such an impact on me that I was able to wear my brace on the outside of my clothes for the first time on the flight back to the UK. As an added bonus, during those three days at the convention, I met some of my greatest friends. The best part is that I'm still friends with all of them today.

I'm now 16 years old and I no longer wear my back brace, but believe it or not, I was reluctant to give it up! It had become a part of me and a part I was proud of. I'm also forever thankful for the Scoliosis SOS Clinic; they gave me a sense of hope and showed me that with strength and determination you can prove anyone wrong. With the clinic's help, my curvature improved to 48°, which was a massive achievement. I'm also motivated to continue doing my physiotherapy, as I now understand that scoliosis is life-long.

Today, I lead the Curvy Girls' chapter for England and hope to help more and more girls overcome the challenges of scoliosis. I'm so thankful for Curvy Girls, because if you had told me three years ago that not only would I be confident in having scoliosis, but that I could stand up and deliver a talk about it (or even write my story in a book) I wouldn't have believed you.

Over the years, I have learned that who we are is determined by the challenges we face and the obstacles we overcome. I feel like I've come a long way. The girl who once went through great lengths to hide her brace, no longer needs to hide. I now have the confidence to wear my hair shorter and, on some days, even in a bun.

Scoliosis has been an obstacle, but if it hadn't been for this condition, I wouldn't have confronted my insecurities and learned how to overcome them. One of my insecurities was feeling as if I did not fit in or was not "normal." It took me a while to realize that being normal can come in many different forms and having scoliosis is definitely one of them— It was my kind of normal.

While my journey certainly isn't over, I know that whatever happens I'll be able to get through it. And to anyone out there who is struggling, I promise that you will get through it all, too!

WHERE ALYSSA IS TODAY

Today Alyssa continues her physiotherapy and is a wonderful role model for the girls in her support group. She attributes her passion to study medicine to her experience with Curvy Girls.

Coping with scoliosis has helped Alyssa see the importance of addressing the emotional impact of a physical condition. She plans to use this awareness in her approach to medicine.

Hope House

Jusna

I think my story is above all one of hope, and applies to any kind of crisis in life. Though this period in Alyssa's life was challenging at times, we never lost hope that things would get better.

Hope House was the name of the main building in Alyssa's primary school. It is a gorgeous Georgian mansion on the hills of Bath, England, and held so many happy memories of those early years for Alyssa and us as a family. Each time we drive past, we recall those fond memories that this building holds. It was a magical, happy time in Alyssa's life.

As a young child, Alyssa's passion and enthusiasm for life shone like a beacon. She never complained about anything, was always up for new experiences and was eager to please and help others. This was perhaps a legacy of being suddenly taken ill at six months old due to being given the wrong childhood vaccine at a routine appointment. Alyssa nearly died; she was in intensive care, and in and out of hospital, until the age of three. Perhaps as a result, she was determined to be the most active child who embraced everyone and everything that life had to offer. Alyssa was, and still is, my little miracle.

Life was good and the desperate memories of her early years faded away until one cold winter afternoon in December. Alyssa was twelve years old, and we had plans to do some shopping after her hockey match at school. We were also looking forward to hosting our extended family from Scotland for Christmas, and Alyssa was quite excited. But when I picked her up after school that day, Alyssa looked downcast and not her usual happy self. She said her back hurt and that she was in some pain, but still wanted to do her shopping. We went into the centre of Bath, a city built on hills that invariably means quite a bit of walking uphill and down. After the first shop, we walked downhill for about six minutes. By the time we got to the local department store, she was in so much pain she decided to lie down flat on the floor in the children's section and did not care what anyone thought of her. It was clear that she was in severe pain, and I started to worry about what could be wrong with her.

Alyssa had been complaining about back pain on and off for a few weeks—but nothing that made me think there was something seriously wrong. I had already made an appointment for her to see our family doctor between Christmas and New Years. But it was a busy time of year with lots of holiday activities, and Alyssa did not wish to give up her free time to see the doctor. I, too, was not unduly worried at the time since Alyssa was very active and lived for the various sports she played competitively; I truly thought her pain was from overexertion.

But as I saw her lying on the floor in the department store, I knew that this was something more serious. My fears were compounded when she recovered enough to get up and try on a jumpsuit. As she turned around with her long hair tied up, I noticed a large lump on her right shoulder. Staring at her back, I did not know what to make of the lump. I thought that she may have inadvertently left a piece of tissue paper in the clothing so I asked her to remove any packaging that she might have missed. She checked and said there was nothing there. I did not say anything but went into the changing room with her to get a closer look at her bare back. I was shocked to see her right shoulder blade protruding significantly, forming a large mass. The color drained from my face but I tried to keep calm.

FEARING THE WORST

Due to Alyssa's past medical history, I suspected something very serious might be wrong, perhaps a cancerous tumor. Childhood leukemia crossed my mind as that was a possibility that she had previously been tested for. I spent that evening on the internet and did come across scoliosis, but as I had never heard of it before, I was not so sure. With the Christmas holidays upon us, I realized it would be difficult to see any specialist sooner than the appointment I had already made with our general practitioner. But luckily my husband happened to have a physiotherapy appointment in two days. We agreed that he would take Alyssa with him for his treatment and also to seek advice as she was still in pain. The physiotherapist confirmed straight away that he suspected she had scoliosis. He recommended a clinic in London, which specialized in scoliosis treatment. Alyssa's pain was getting worse and within days she could barely walk longer than 15 minutes. We tried to keep things normal for the festive period but inside I was breaking apart with fright; my active daughter could barely walk. I managed to get an appointment with the London clinic a few days after Christmas. I prayed for her condition to be something that could be cured. The doctors did a thermal scan of Alyssa's back and confirmed that she had a double curvature scoliosis. They were confident that with intensive specific physiotherapy treatment and continued physiotherapy she could be pain-free. They recommended a spinal surgeon to confirm the diagnosis and craft a treatment plan.

Things moved at a pace, and we booked Alyssa in for two weeks of intensive physiotherapy treatment at the clinic for late January. Meanwhile, the whole medical process started. We saw our family doctor, the wonderful Dr. Brenda Nye and she confirmed that Alyssa had scoliosis. In the UK you need to be referred to a specialist by your general practitioner, or GP. Dr. Nye, characteristically did all she could to help and referred Alyssa to the consultant we wanted. Without her help and support the whole process in those early years would have been far worse.

NO EMPATHY OR COMPASSION

The first consultant surgeon, who was supposedly an expert in childhood scoliosis, left his empathy and compassion elsewhere when we had our meeting with him. Alyssa and I were visibly shocked by the X-ray and sat ashen-faced as the surgeon matter-of-factly confirmed that Alyssa had a spinal curvature of 56°. Because Alyssa was a teen and in a rapid growth period, he believed that the spinal curve could get much worse and Alyssa's condition could continue to deteriorate. He recommended spinal surgery by that summer. His words drifted over me as I tried to look away from his computer screen and Alyssa's X-ray. I went into autopilot and kept asking questions and cross-examining what he said, trying to find some hope or even some alternate treatment. None was forthcoming and the consultation quickly came to an end. I was stunned and searched for words to help comfort my daughter.

"So, this doctor is saying that I have to have surgery now, which may not work and will mean that I probably won't ever do any of the sports I do now," Alyssa said after we left his office. "And if I don't go ahead with surgery, I will be in so much more pain that I would not be able to do anything anyway. Surgery could mean that I may end up immobile; without surgery, I would be in pain and possibly in a wheelchair too!"

"Well," she continued, "I am not accepting any of these options. He is wrong and wrong again, and I am certainly not going to cry, and you won't cry either."

Alyssa was trying valiantly but failing to fight back her tears in defiance. I looked at my 12-year-old daughter, and belying her slight frame, saw such strength of character and determination. Yet at the same time she was so vulnerable, with her eyes pleading in desperation for help to find some other solution. It was too much for me; I made excuses and went to the lady's room to cry. It was then I decided that I would do all that was possible to help Alyssa become pain-free and still be herself, without surgery.

INTENSIVE PHYSIOTHERAPY

Alyssa took two weeks out of school to attend a scoliosis clinic in London. The clinic specializes in specific and intensive physiotherapy for patients with scoliosis, using the principles of the Schroth Method along with the concepts of other therapies. Since each patient has a different curve pattern, an exercise program is tailored just for them. The idea behind learning these scoliosis-specific exercises is so patients with severe scoliosis can lead pain-free lives, and possibly avoid surgery. However, since scoliosis is a lifelong condition, the patient must be committed to their program to ensure the healthiest spine outcome.

The physiotherapy from 9 a.m. to 5 p.m. everyday left her physically exhausted. But by the end of it she was no longer in severe pain. She was given a program tailored for her to do 45 minutes of exercise each day. Then came multiple hospital trips for X-rays, MRI scans and so on. We found a different consultant who understood Alyssa better and had at least some bedside manner. He offered a similar diagnosis, but encouragingly found Alyssa's balance to be perfect as she was now mostly pain-free. He suggested that we could try a combination of bracing and exercise for the next few years, monitor the progression of the curve until Alyssa stopped growing—and hold off on doing any surgery.

Alyssa was fitted with a plastic back brace that she would have to wear 23 hours a day, at least during the initial period. At first, she hated it, partly because of the pain and discomfort from the device. And then there was the issue of how it made her look. She could hardly wear anything normal over it. Alyssa was usually a compliant child, but now she kicked up a fuss and pleaded not to have to wear it. However, her father and I were equally determined that she should wear the brace. We both knew that the alternative was surgery, which we were determined to avoid. My husband, Andrew, was much better at this enforcement than I was. He did not give in to any emotional outbursts or pleading and, unlike me, never relented. Alyssa had never seen this rigid, unbending, side of her father. When it came to wearing her brace and doing her exercises, he became more akin to a sergeant major than her loving father.

DAD'S NEW ROLE

"I felt conflicted. I was always the 'fun' parent, the indulgent one who would let the girls get away with breaking the rules," Andrew said. "Sometimes I'd team up with them, joining in some light-hearted subterfuge to hide minor indiscretions from Jusna. But circumstances changed with Alyssa's diagnosis—and I had to change, too."

This new state of affairs was not easy for either Andrew or Alyssa. She had a very close relationship with her father, secure in the knowledge that there was nothing he would not do for her. I knew, too, that Andrew would do anything to protect his children and keep them from harm; in Alyssa's case fate had added a twist to that primal instinct. In order to protect Alyssa, Andrew would often have to go against her wishes. It was all very counterintuitive; instead of reaching out and comforting his daughter, he was forcing her to do the very thing (wear the brace/exercise) that was causing her distress.

"I worried that I was being too strict with Alyssa," Andrew said. "And I worried that I might be harming our relationship. But it was a risk I had to take. I feared that if she didn't stick with her treatment plan, we could confront an unsuccessful outcome that would put her future well-being in jeopardy."

PUSHBACK

Both Andrew and I suspected that there was more to Alyssa's dislike of her brace than just her complaints that it was unsightly and uncomfortable.

The antipathy towards her brace and treatment was her way of pushing back against her condition. By not accepting her treatment, she was being defiant against the whole situation. Andrew and I believed that it was important for Alyssa to accept her condition and learn to live with it.

In time, Alyssa did, indeed, learn to live with scoliosis along with the brace, and her relationship with her father evolved along the way. They are perhaps closer today than they were before. As time went by and Alyssa got older, Andrew backed off from his tough "Sergeant Major" role. Instead, he volunteered to go with her when she went to do her physiotherapy exercises and did some of them right alongside her. Andrew and Alyssa wound up spending a lot of time together—and in doing so Alyssa gained a deep insight into to her father's rather eclectic taste in music. She became educated in whole genres that she would otherwise never have encountered.

One of the most difficult things to accept when you have a child with a chronic condition is that the condition is here to stay, today, tomorrow, and well into the future. Even when your rational mind realizes that there is no magic cure, there remains a vestige of hope that your child's condition will eventually become so negligible that it has little or no impact on their lives.

In order to help your child, not only do you begin to explore and devour everything you can to learn about the latest developments and treatments for their condition, but you look into practical ways to make their everyday lives as normal as possible. And so it was with Andrew and me. We examined and dug into what Alyssa could and could not do at school, what she could wear and so forth. Each new situation would need careful adjustment. Fortunately, Alyssa's school and teachers were very supportive and made allowances for her. Alyssa was a popular child and having been there for everyone, her close friends were initially there for her, too. She coped with school, but didn't want everyone to know that she had scoliosis or wore a brace.

"I don't want to be defined by my condition," Alyssa said. She would go to elaborate lengths to hide her brace, everything from wearing baggy clothes to growing her hair long in order to cover the protrusion at the back.

MENTAL STRAIN TAKES A TOLL

After the initial diagnosis, we got into a routine with the many medical and physical issues arising from scoliosis, which lasted about two years. But then, the mental strain of coping with being different started to take its toll on Alyssa. Increasingly, she could not take part in activities both in and out of school. As a result, Alyssa suddenly began to be excluded from her friendship groups, all because of her scoliosis. My once happy child gradually became withdrawn and hated how she looked and felt. Alyssa became increasingly depressed but refused to talk to me about it.

It is hard to watch your child suffer both mentally and physically. I knew that she did not want to speak to me; it was her way of coping and I did not want to force her. She was happiest at home with her siblings, who never changed their attitudes and feelings towards her. Like any siblings, they could annoy her intensely at times—but they were also a source of comfort as only siblings could be.

If there's one piece of advice I can give, it is this: If you have a child with a chronic condition, it is important to treat them as normally as possible. Alyssa's siblings fulfilled that role with aplomb. Beyond some practical help, they made no allowances for her scoliosis. Her younger brother Matthias would demand that she play games with him and do all the things that they always did together, making it hard for Alyssa to withdraw too much into herself. It was in being treated so normally by them, to my mind, that helped Alyssa cope. Nevertheless, coping with everyday practicalities and feeling different started to affect Alyssa's emotional state.

One day she broke down and cried, telling me how hard the last couple of years had been for her. She told me how she would hide in a bathroom at school so she did not have to walk in to assembly in front of the other students. Her brace made a noise that everyone could hear when she walked into the quiet hall, and she felt everyone would stare at her. She did not want to tell me because she feared I would have gone to school officials and obtained permission for her to waive the events. And for Alyssa, that would have meant standing out. She told me, too, how people knocked on her brace and laughed at her; again, she knew I would try and resolve those things.

POWERLESS TO HELP

"Only you can't make things better this time Mummy, can you?" she asked. "I will still have scoliosis and still have to wear the brace. I have to live with this, and so I want to do it in my own way." I felt at once heartbroken and helpless but knew she was right. Although Alyssa still had individual friends who were kind to her, she felt that nobody understood what she was going through, except perhaps her elder sister, Octavia.

Octavia came to me one day and said, "What Alyssa needs is to talk to someone, preferably someone who has had something similar to her, or a counselor." She had found a support group that Martha Hunt, the supermodel, was part of called Curvy Girls. It was based in the USA but she was sure we could find a similar group in England. Unfortunately, there was no group like it in England. Octavia and Alyssa then sought to learn more about Curvy Girls and they liked what they found. Octavia suggested that Alyssa contact Curvy Girls to inquire about setting up a new chapter here in England. I was a little skeptical. I did not want Alyssa to have much more to do, or to take on other people's problems when she was suffering herself. But Octavia was certain she was right. She said that if there was anyone who could help others, it was Alyssa—and she needed to do this. Alyssa, too, believed that it was the right step to take. She said she had struggled for years feeling so isolated, and if she could help just one person not to feel the way she did, that it would help her feel better. I agreed for Alyssa to apply to become a leader for Curvy Girls. It was one of the best decisions I have ever made.

A NEW ATTITUDE

Joining Curvy Girls completely transformed Alyssa's attitude toward her condition. Within months of setting up the English Chapter of Curvy Girls in July 2018, Alyssa and I were traveling to New York for our first biennial Conference hosted by the Curvy Girls Scoliosis Foundation. There, we met and talked to people who had similar experiences to Alyssa. Suddenly, it seemed that the whole world had scoliosis. Alyssa started to smile again; she realized that scoliosis would no longer define her. Instead, the group empowered her to not allow the condition to rob her of her happiness. For the first time since her diagnosis, a burden was lifted and she no longer needed to hide her scoliosis.

When we flew back home to England, she wore her brace for the first time on the outside of her clothing. I was so proud of her! During the last two years, Alyssa has taken her new role as a Curvy Girls' leader very seriously, and worked hard to promote awareness of scoliosis and the organization. She began to educate others about scoliosis by doing numerous presentations on scoliosis. She posted pictures of her X-rays online, and she showed them as part of her talks on scoliosis. Alyssa is now 16 and has been brace-free for several months. She will be monitored for another two years, until she is 18, to see whether she will require surgery. But as of now, the combination of the brace and exercises have been successful.

Today, Alyssa is an advocate for scoliosis and maintains a positive but pragmatic outlook. It is a truism that altruism has double benefits. Alyssa joined Curvy Girls to help others and, in her endeavors to help others, she was helped herself. Whether she requires surgery or not, having come through that period where the future looked quite bleak, I know that whatever happens Alyssa will come through it. Whatever she does, as her mother, I am proud of all she has done so far and grateful that we found Curvy Girls in time to help her to become herself again.

Part 1: Memoirs

Jamiah

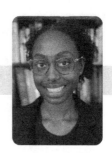

Meet Jamiah from Connecticut

Age: 22

Spinal Fusion Surgery at age 14

Jamiah loves to spend time with loved ones, listen to music, travel and exercise. One of her favorite things to do is teach spin classes.

Curvy Girls has shown Jamiah the power of a supportive community.

Jamiah was never given the opportunity to wear a brace; surgery was her only option.

Having watched the HALO Awards a year prior to her diagnosis, she secretly admired the person who started a support group for girls with scoliosis. Jamiah never would have expected that this would be her story too.

Jamiah's Message: Please know that there is strength in all of your voices. I encourage each of you to use yours to advocate for yourself, especially when it comes to your body and overall health.

Jamiah Bennett and her mother, Cynthia Parker

The Power Within

"Out of your darkest moments, you find your greatest strengths"

—Anonymous

Jamiah: "You'll have to have surgery," were the words I was not expecting to hear. My heart started racing so fast I thought it was going to pop out of my chest. I looked over at my mom as tears began to well up in my eyes. I could feel my body slowly starting to shrink as I collapsed into my own lap.

Mom: When the doctor said those words, we were both in shock. One look at Jamiah's face and I knew I could not react the way I felt. I had to stay strong as it was quite apparent Jamiah was very upset.

Jamiah: "What happened to wearing a brace?" is what I wanted to say, but I couldn't. Instead, I just sat there frozen and yet everything was happening at record speed. I remembered hearing the doctor say I have scoliosis. It was a word I was familiar with since both my mom and grandmother were diagnosed when they were around my age.

Mom: It was the scoliosis screening I had asked for that led us to this appointment with an orthopedic specialist. I first discovered Jamiah had a curved spine when I was styling her hair. I noticed she wasn't standing straight, so I asked her to bend over, and that's when I saw the lump on her back. Devastated, I asked her to request an early screening for scoliosis from her school nurse. But I was pretty sure I knew what I was looking at; I'd been there, too.

Jamiah: Even though I knew what scoliosis was, I just never fully processed what it might mean for me—or the medical treatment plan that inevitably came along with the diagnosis. As far as treatment, all I knew was that some people had to wear a hard plastic brace for a certain number of hours a day in an effort to stop their spine from curving. That's it. That is the only form of treatment I had ever heard of—a plastic brace that you wear for a few hours a day. But then the doctor showed me the black and white X-ray of my "C" shaped spine with a 45° curve. I just stared at the X-ray in complete disbelief. It wasn't until that moment that I realized the true impact that scoliosis can have on a spine.

Mom: I never would have imagined that Jamiah's scoliosis would be this serious. No one ever told me that scoliosis could be hereditary. And I couldn't understand why her scoliosis would be any different from what my mother and I experienced; both of us had had a mild curve that didn't require any treatment. I was so confused and overwhelmed.

Jamiah: We walked out of the orthopedist's office in a daze, holding a referral to a local orthopedic surgeon. I could not wrap my mind around the fact that I had no options other than surgery. Going into the appointment, I knew there was a strong possibility I had scoliosis, like my mother and grandmother, but never did I expect my journey to be so different than theirs.

Mom: I have to be honest, not knowing what the surgery entailed saved me from myself.

My mind was all over the place. I was so overwhelmed and the last thing I wanted to do is allow Jamiah to see my anxiety.

Do I talk about what we just heard, or do we sit in silence? I took a deep breath and told her in the most confident voice, "We will get through this." It's the only thing I could think of saying, because if I said anything else, I couldn't guarantee I wouldn't become emotional. And the last thing I wanted Jamiah to see was me being upset. My only goal after hearing "surgery" was to be supportive and strong for Jamiah.

Jamiah: I stepped into the car slowly bringing one foot in at a time as I focused on holding back the same tears that started to form in the doctor's office. Trying to process what I just heard, I realized that I did not want everyone at my school to know about this diagnosis. But I did want my best friend to know. I made her promise, as eighth graders do, not to tell any other person in our school. It had to stay between us because I was nervous about what people would think. Everyone in school knew what scoliosis was because we all had to get screened. Looking back, there were probably others kids my age diagnosed with scoliosis; I just did not want to be the first person to say that I had it. I was devastated by the news and didn't know how to react.

Mom: Over the next few weeks I could clearly see that Jamiah was very nervous about having surgery to correct her scoliosis; we all were. And then one day everything seemed to get a little easier when Jamiah had a flashback of a show she remembered that highlighted a girl who had scoliosis.

Jamiah: About a year prior to my diagnosis, I remembered sitting in the living room with my whole family watching a show on TeenNick called the HALO Awards, which featured stories about teens "Helping And Leading Others." I was fascinated by all of the amazing things these teenagers, who were around my age, were doing in the world. I was particularly intrigued by one girl who had started a group for girls with scoliosis. I could not remember her name or the name of her organization. All I could remember was that I thought she was really cool. After all, she was surprised by Nick Cannon at her high school and got to hang out with Justin Timberlake, all because she started this amazing support group.

Mom: I was so happy that Jamiah remembered this show. It was great seeing her get excited about something again. She was now on a new mission to learn all about this girl and her group. It definitely helped her feel better knowing this girl had scoliosis too, that she'd gone through surgery, and was doing just fine.

Jamiah: I wasn't able to remember the name of the girl from the HALO awards, so I went to the quickest resource I knew—the internet. Within thirty seconds, I found the cool girl's name and the name of her organization: Leah Stoltz and Curvy Girls. I was overwhelmed with joy because I knew this group would be able to provide me with the support I needed during this time.

Little did I know the people I would meet in the Curvy Girls' organization would support me way beyond what I could have ever imagined.

Mom: Jamiah's focus and determination to find this group was nonstop. If Curvy Girls could help her feel less alone and not let her think about her upcoming surgery day and night, we were all for it. In the interim, I needed to have Jamiah's younger sister, Asha, checked for scoliosis, now that I knew this condition can be passed on from generation to generation.

I wasn't able to prevent Jamiah's surgery, but I could make sure Asha had a fighting chance to avoid surgery if we monitored her more closely.

Jamiah: When I came across the Curvy Girls' website, I tried to find a chapter near me so I could start attending on a regular basis. Unfortunately, the closest group to me turned out to be in Brooklyn, New York which was about two hours away from my home in southern Connecticut. While the distance wasn't too bad, it was not feasible for my family to drive every month. So, I reached out to the leader of that chapter and we worked out a plan so I could Skype into their monthly meetings. Although I never physically attended a meeting, those hour-long conversations with girls who were experiencing something similar to me were some of the best conversations I had during this time. Thanks to Curvy Girls, I eventually came to embrace and understand my scoliosis.

I gradually became so comfortable with my condition that I did not mind if people knew about it. In fact, I encouraged discussions about scoliosis and my experience with it. One of the first people I spoke with, outside of my family and best friends, was my school nurse. Remember when I thought I would be the first one in my school with scoliosis? It turns out that I wasn't. The nurse told me that there was another girl in the school that also had surgery and she could connect her with me. The nurse reached out to the girl's family and a few days later I was in touch with that student!

Mom: Jamiah and I were very appreciative that the schoolgirl's family agreed to meet with us. They answered so many questions and also referred us to their surgeon, Dr. Mark Lee, from the Connecticut Children's Medical Center, for a second opinion. After meeting with Dr. Lee, I felt less anxiety as he was very detail-oriented and supportive. He had an amazing bedside manner and I appreciated how he communicated with Jamiah—he spoke directly to her. But what completely sold me about Dr. Lee was when he gave Jamiah his personal cell phone number. He said, "You can contact me with any questions or concerns." It was at that moment I knew we found our surgeon.

Jamiah: I was nervous meeting Dr. Lee, but by the end of that appointment I felt very comfortable with him. He made himself available to answer all of my questions, even if it was after office hours.

But what truly helped me the most was being able to talk to my friend in school and my group of Curvy Girls' peers. I could talk freely about so many issues relating to my upcoming surgery, and that was exactly what I needed. The conversations made me feel understood in a way that my family and friends couldn't. Don't get me wrong, I am grateful to be able to say that my family and friends were incredibly supportive throughout my journey; however, the support from Curvy Girls was on a whole other level.

Mom: Curvy Girls seemed to be exactly what Jamiah needed at this time. As a family we were committed to being as supportive as possible. That was our goal. We couldn't have asked more from Asha, who never acted out or complained about the extra attention that Jamiah was getting. She did whatever she could to help her older sister—which was wonderful to witness especially since she was six years younger.

Jamiah: My surgery was set for October 11th. Somehow having an exact date made this very real. I became more nervous, although I tried to hide it. I kind of wish I stopped Googling spinal fusion surgeries on the internet because all it did was make me more nervous. While all surgeries are serious, spinal surgery seemed to be on a different level. Reading all this just made things worse, which led to more anxiety and fear. I kept thinking, how was it that I was headed to surgery less than a year after being diagnosed.

Mom: The night before her surgery Jamiah was very quiet, which was to be expected. I continued to try to remain calm for Jamiah, which ironically helped me. Periodically, I would remind Jamiah what an amazing doctor we had, hoping to distract her from any negative or fearful thoughts. Still, nothing was going to completely release the underlying nerves we were all feeling that night. I'm not sure if it was right or wrong but I kept reminding myself not to say too much. Act normal was my mantra.

Jamiah: The morning of the surgery we had to get up before sunrise. We had an early morning appointment and a 45-minute drive to the hospital. My nerves started to get to me, but I held it all in. Maybe I thought it would help me get through this better if I didn't cry or let anyone see how truly scared I was.

Mom: When it was time to go down to the operating room Jamiah got really quiet, which really upset me because I knew what she was going through. I hated feeling so helpless. I knew she was scared, and I couldn't do anything to help her feel better. When the nurse said only one person could go with her into the operating room, I immediately said it would be me.

I held her hand as we walked down the hospital corridor toward the O.R. I wanted to cry so badly but knew I had to be strong for her. When a doctor administered the general anesthesia, she started shaking and I freaked out! The doctor said it was because she was fighting the drugs and that she didn't want to be put to sleep. That is when I started crying. I couldn't help her, and I felt even worse because I knew she needed me.

Jamiah: I thought I could hold it together until I actually had to let go of my mom's hands. I remembered being super cold and my body starting to shake. The next thing I remembered I was waking up in the recovery room.

Mom: I was not prepared at all when her anesthesia wore off and she woke up. They kept telling her to breathe. I asked what was going on. Was she not breathing on her own? She was, and apparently this was all routine. Still, that moment freaked me out. Jamiah's face was also very swollen. I later learned that that, too, was a normal reaction from lying on her stomach the entire five hours of surgery. I definitely was not prepared for that either. Knowledge is power and I wish I had been better prepared that day.

Jamiah: The recovery was certainly a challenge I will never forget. I struggled trying to get used to my "new body" after surgery. Everything felt so stiff and my back would itch but I wasn't able to scratch it. I remember needing to go to the bathroom but having to wait for a nurse to come help me get up because I couldn't move on my own. I remember attempting to take my first step on a flat surface and then taking my first step going upstairs.

I will never take my ability to walk for granted ever again. Despite the challenges and hardships the surgery presented to me physically and mentally, I learned a lot of valuable lessons from those recovery days that I can apply to my life today and for years to come.

Mom: Jamiah's surgery was a complete success, but the recovery was very painful for her. When we got her home, she had a lot of trouble moving on her own. She needed assistance with every move, including going to the bathroom and showering. Parents need to be prepared for those first few weeks after surgery because their children will be heavily dependent on them night and day. I had to turn Jamiah from one side to the other every two hours. For six weeks there were many sleepless nights for both of us, but I didn't care. I would do anything to get her better. As far as I was concerned, I had one job and that was to make her as happy and comfortable as possible during her recovery—while not letting her know that I was burnt out both mentally and physically.

Jamiah: As soon as I began getting stronger, my first thoughts were about helping that next girl with their scoliosis journey. My conversations with the student at my school and my experiences with Curvy Girls' meetings galvanized me into finding a community of scoliosis patients closer to home. I reached out to Leah's mom, Robin, to inquire about starting a Curvy Girls' chapter in my home state, Connecticut. Robin was very receptive to the idea. Not long after and only one year after the airing of the HALO Awards, Curvy Girls of Connecticut was formed. I was ecstatic.

Mom: Starting this group was exactly what Jamiah needed. I believe it actually fueled her recovery. Taking on this new role as a leader seemed like the perfect fit for Jamiah. It was so great to see her smiling and making plans for future activities with Curvy Girls. Jamiah was happy.

Jamiah: I remember my first meeting as if it were yesterday. Robin and Leah crossed the Long Island Sound by ferry from New York to my home in Connecticut to support me for my first meeting. I could not believe that the girl I had seen on the TeenNick HALO Awards only a year earlier was coming to my house! Leah was the girl who started this community and she was taking time to come see me start mine. I was beyond honored.

Mom: Jamiah proudly led her group until she graduated from high school. Through her involvement with Curvy Girls she has made many lifelong friendships. I am so proud of Jamiah because she didn't become a victim of her scoliosis, but instead became victorious. She championed through the difficult times and persevered on a path to help others.

Jamiah: When I was first told I had scoliosis and would require surgery, I thought my life would never be the same. I thought I would not be able to enjoy life the way I use to. I was partly right. Being diagnosed with scoliosis and having surgery did change my life. It hasn't been the same but not in the way I feared. I have grown tremendously—my confidence has increased, my ability to empathize is greater, and my drive to help others while helping myself has become a big part of my identity. I will forever be grateful for my scoliosis diagnosis and the experiences it led me to, including becoming the first Curvy Girls' Leader of CT.

At the time of that first meeting, little did I know that I would remain in that position until I went off to college. Handing over that Curvy Girls' position was one of the hardest things I have ever done. Emotionally, I felt like I was giving up part of my identity. But I also knew the chapter was in great hands with our new leader, Julianne.

Mom: Sometimes things happen in our lives that we have no control over. Scoliosis is one of them.

Try not to allow the diagnosis to overwhelm you, like it did for me. I wish I was given more options at Jamiah's initial diagnosis. I felt so alone and didn't have anyone to turn to. However, today things are so different. Families worldwide have a wonderful resource to reach out to because of Curvy Girls. If you are newly diagnosed and are thinking of seeking a second and third opinion, you should do it. And if you are not sure where to go, I hope you look for the nearest Curvy Girls' chapter or email the Foundation directly for additional support.

Jamiah: For some girls, scoliosis is the first curveball that life throws at us. Initially we are scared, angry, frustrated, confused, and naturally, we cry. I want you to know it's okay if you experience one of those emotions or all of them. I actually think it's healthier for us to acknowledge what we are feeling rather than pretending we are fine all the time. Once we allow ourselves to face our biggest fears, the sooner we will be able to release it and move forward. This new-found strength will fuel you to not only become the warrior you were meant to be, but it will provide you with lifelong skills way beyond your scoliosis years.

WHERE JAMIAH IS TODAY

Shortly after she stepped down as a leader of the Connecticut Chapter, she was invited to become part of Curvy Girls Mentor initiative, which allows seasoned leaders to use their experience to train new leaders. She has also served as the Coordinator of Diversity, Equity, and Inclusion. In these roles, she is able to apply what she learned through her journalism and sociology studies at her alma mater, the University of Connecticut—verbal and written communication, understanding of various groups and perspectives, and analyzing how societal events impact people. In the fall of 2021, she will be attending the University of Pennsylvania Graduate School of Education Independent School Teaching Residency program where she will pursue a career in secondary education.

Katelyn

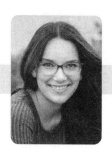

Meet Katelyn from Iowa

Age: 19

Braced at age 13

Ended treatment age 17

Katelyn loves reading, being with family and spending time outdoors.

Being in Curvy Girls provided Katelyn with a community of people who have an intimate understanding of each other's struggles—to literally walk in each other's braces and share the same scars.

Katelyn's diagnosis made her angry all the time. She felt lost, and completely alone until she read, Straight Talk with the Curvy Girls. Being able to relate to the other girls in the book became Katelyn's lifeline for hope.

Katelyn's Message: At the beginning of my scoliosis journey, all I wanted was to change my diagnosis. Now, I wouldn't give up my scoliosis or my scoliosis journey for anything.

Katelyn Winkler and her mother, Amy Winkler

Twisted Road to Acceptance

Katelyn

I received a card in the mail from a distant relative. It had a few words of encouragement with a vague greeting card message about perseverance. I threw it in the trash. I didn't feel very strong or perseverant; I felt angry. Fiery, all-consuming, exhaustive anger at the betrayal of my body.

The summer before seventh grade I was in the doctor's office with my mom for my annual checkup. We both expected that it would be routine, mundane, and altogether quite without circumstance. The only exciting element was the new, electronic patient history database my doctor had begun to use. That meant that my mom had to fill out still another medical history form. But there was one item that she forgot to jot down on the form—my grandmother had scoliosis. She made it a point to verbally tell the doctor when he walked into the exam room.

In the exam room, the doctor decided to first check my spine and started pressing along my back, counting vertebrae while simultaneously listening to my heart with his stethoscope. Abruptly he stopped listening and started feeling my spine more closely. The hairs on my neck prickled and my palms started to sweat. I couldn't hear anything except the low drone of background noise in the office.

"What's going on?" I asked the doctor. He and Mom had begun to engage in an exuberant conversation about this word, scoliosis. They both seemed to be aware of what the word meant. Words like surgery and X-rays, along with my name, were thrown around. I begged someone to explain to me what was going on, but the only answer was the continual crescendo of a buzzing in my ears.

STARTING SEVENTH GRADE WITH SCOLIOSIS

That day I walked out with both a referral to see an orthopedist and an uneasy mind. I had been diagnosed with a 27° scoliosis curve just days before the start of seventh grade.

I was confused, uncertain, and the internet was plaguing my mind with 100+ degree-curves, horror stories of surgery gone wrong, and unlikely scenarios that left me wondering if I was going to end up paralyzed. Until now, I had a clean bill of health. This was the first time I had ever experienced a doctor's appointment in which the end result was a diagnosis. Scoliosis. The word felt foreign as it rolled off my tongue. I couldn't quite swallow the reality of what was happening to me. I vividly remember just wanting to understand.

My first orthopedic appointment is a blurry memory. What I do remember is that he made me feel small. He laughed at my tears and joked that my life was over. After the appointment I wanted to crawl in a hole and never leave.

In the waiting room of my first orthotist's office there was a bird. I couldn't help but laugh at the irony of the cage it sat in. At that time, I felt that my own cage was waiting for me in the room.

FIRST LOOK

I had never seen a brace before that day. No one had shown me any pictures or given me any idea of what it would look like. As the orthotist brought it in, I got the same feeling you experience when the rollercoaster drops a hundred feet down. It was so much bulkier and cumbersome than I had anticipated.

When I was finally expected to put it on, I didn't feel as though it was my body anymore.

> I felt as if the real me was floating somewhere in the room, screaming, but no one could hear me.

I was screaming for someone to let me out, but all I could do was watch my own hands tighten the straps further. I was the bird and the person who caged it.

Two months later I felt like I was going insane. I couldn't catch a breath, probably because the brace was squeezing me so tightly, but also because, emotionally, I was spinning out of control.

On a blustery fall day, I saw my second orthopedist, Dr. Weinstein. My parents and I held our breath as we navigated our way a couple hours across the state to the new hospital. After my brutal first visit with an orthopedist who demonstrated no sense of care or concern for his patient, I was determined not to let my guard down or expect too much from this new doctor.

Even finding his office in a large complex was tricky. There were multiple floors and lots of turns along the way—all of which seemed to raise the tension for us even more. But when we arrived, we were immediately taken care of. I was whisked from the check-in desk to another waiting area where a kind nurse helped me fill out an online quiz about all my symptoms.

> This was the first time any of the doctors, nurses, and staff ever inquired about the pain I was experiencing physically and emotionally.

It felt like a good omen, and I hoped that the rest of my visit would be positive, too.

A CARING ATTITUDE

We sat for a long time, waiting to go in for the specialized X-ray images that would tell the doctor more about my case, and I could feel myself getting tense wondering what was going to happen next. But then, the most kind and outgoing technician, Randall, came into the waiting room to meet me. He accompanied me on the short walk to a room housing the giant orange machine used for taking EOS images, which is a low-dose, weight-bearing X-ray technology that can simultaneously take full-body, frontal, and side-view images of the skeletal system. The device is less risky to the patient than some other technologies because it uses far less radiation. Randall's quiet and supportive demeanor made all the difference in my experience. Any thought of fear had left my mind long ago.

My inner sense of calm continued as I met with Dr. Weinstein for the first time and found him warm and welcoming—just like his staff. My parents were at ease, too, especially after hearing that he had recently published a study in the prestigious New England Journal of Medicine concluding that bracing is effective in scoliosis treatment. When I walked out of that appointment with a prescription for a brace, I felt excited, knowing this time it would be different. Later, I nicknamed him 'Dr. Fluffy Bunny' because of his white hair and calm, warm presence.

Although I was initially hopeful, the brace was still a difficult adjustment to say the least. Nonchalantly, I told my closest friends about it, hoping they wouldn't find it a big deal if I didn't make it seem like one. Yet, inside I was still yearning for someone who could truly understand me.

The first day I wore my brace to school I felt an overwhelming urge to curl up in the bathroom and never leave. Begrudgingly, I walked into the classroom and took my books out of my locker. I tried to put them on the ground to retrieve more supplies from the back of the locker but immediately realized that I couldn't bend enough to reach the floor. My brace kept me locked in a distinctly unfriendly embrace. A tear rolled down my cheek, but I shook it off. The rest of the morning went at a turtle's pace.

BETRAYAL

Finally, when I reached my vocabulary class, I could take a deep breath because my friends were there. When I sat down at the table, I smiled at them and we started working. It was back to a normal day and my nervousness slipped away—at least for a moment. Then, my best friend since elementary school hissed cruel words to me during a trivial disagreement. "I will tell everyone about your brace if you don't do exactly what I say," she said.

It was as if she had slapped me across the face. I was so shocked I didn't have any response. My best friend of five years had just betrayed me in a single instant. It was in that moment I realized how quickly a friendship could dissipate.

Even though I was wearing my plastic shell she had managed to puncture right to my heart. I felt a new kind of anger and a new kind of isolation and hurt.

> The anger was only partly directed at my friend; most of it was directed towards scoliosis and how it had changed everything.

I am a self-proclaimed control addict who always maintained a grip on every aspect of my life. When the asteroid 'scoliosis' hit, it rocked my world in a way I'd never experienced before. I couldn't find my bearings. I felt so angry. I cried and threw tantrums and lashed out at my family. The anger was exhausting, and I cried myself to sleep more times than I ever have in my entire life. More than anything, I felt powerless.

Initially, I believed the worst part of scoliosis would be wearing the brace or having surgery. In that moment I knew, for me, the worst part of scoliosis is how it assumes control over what is supposed to belong to oneself: the body.

FINDING INSPIRATION

Six months after the diagnosis, my thirteenth birthday came. My iciness towards scoliosis had melted a bit and I didn't yell or hide anymore when people talked about scoliosis with me. For my birthday, my mom gave me a book called *Straight Talk with the Curvy Girls*. She knew how much I loved to read, so it was only natural that my scoliosis acceptance story started with a book.

I read it immediately. I couldn't stop reading; I simply couldn't put it down. On page twenty-seven, Rachel wrote, "It's never too late to take back control over your own body." For a Type-A girl like me, this spoke to my soul. Hearing those words, I felt calm and supported. Those nine girls were going through the exact same thing as I was and the idea that I wasn't alone was mind blowing! Heavy and salty tears cascaded down my cheeks like waterfalls of anger and emptiness, finally washing away some of the pain I'd felt for months. I felt the most relief I've ever experienced in my life.

Reading Rachel's words, I knew that in order to accept this diagnosis I had to take back control. And taking back control meant facing my situation with grit, conviction, and confidence.

FIRST CURVY GIRLS' LEADER IN IOWA

A step towards this was becoming the first Curvy Girls Leader of Iowa. I started the group because in my mind helping other girls would heal me. I think the "fake it 'til you make it mantra" appealed to me. If I could even pretend to be strong, perhaps it would eventually come true.

Slowly but surely, I was able to start wearing my brace on the outside of my clothes for everyone to see. I spoke to my classmates and teachers about it without worrying about their reactions. I finally owned my scoliosis.

Doing this required the most strength than I've ever had to muster. Yet, it changed everything for me. I can honestly say that none of this could have been possible without being part of Curvy Girls. Perseverance can completely change the outcome.

> It did not matter if I needed surgery or my curve progressed; the difference between a "bad" outcome and a "good" one was my attitude.

If you are a young girl, newly diagnosed or just had surgery, I want you to know that Curvy Girls is so much more than a group of girls with scoliosis. For me, Curvy Girls has become a network of love and understanding. Curvy Girls is the meeting place of young women who can and want to make a difference in each other's lives. Curvy Girls is about doing it for the next girl, and the next, and the next, so that when another girl is diagnosed, she doesn't have to be alone.

HAVING THE STRENGH TO OVERCOME

To the girl who is reading about my scoliosis journey, I hope you can feel even a fraction of the relief I felt when reading the first edition of *Straight Talk with the Curvy Girls*. I know what it's like to have a friend betray you, have conflict with loved ones, worry about your changing body, and endure hours of doctor's appointments. You *will* get through this, and you will walk away even stronger! If you need someone who understands what you are feeling, please reach out to the nearest Curvy Girls' chapter and attend a meeting.

Now, almost ten years after being diagnosed I have written many pieces about my scoliosis. The striking progression of my emotions and feelings towards scoliosis has always been shown best through my writing. I have written countless diary entries, stories, and even speeches about my scoliosis. I wrote a letter to my first doctor who hurt me. I don't even feel the need to send it. Just by acknowledging my feelings I have been able to memorialize it on paper, where it can no longer weigh me down.

I wrote this poem at the end of seventh grade, almost one year after I was diagnosed. This poem represents how Curvy Girls has changed me.

I glance in the mirror, hesitant.
Resilience prevails
I peel off my brace and
stare.
At the
curved
bent
broken
bruised
pale
Me.
I
see
beauty
strength
powerful
fearlessness.
I see myself staring back at me.

WHERE KATELYN IS TODAY

Today, Katelyn attends the University of Iowa majoring in Sustainability Science with a minor in French. She plans on pursuing higher education and to continue in the area of research throughout her career. Katelyn remains active with Curvy Girls as a Mentor.

It Started With A Book

Amy

It was the end of the summer and time for back-to-school physicals for both of my daughters. My oldest daughter, Katelyn, has some pretty serious anxieties about doctor appointments, so I decided I could only handle taking one girl at a time. I scheduled the two of them on back-to-back days, with Rachel, my youngest, going first. During her visit, the nurse asked for an updated family history. I never like this part because if you're like me your mind goes completely blank. For some reason I can never think of everything on the spot, especially medical issues from my husband's side of the family. That day I did remember an important hereditary condition that I kept forgetting to put on their medical records. Once we got that updated, everything checked out well for Rachel. Whew! A huge relief since she has had various health issues over the years.

Katelyn is my "healthy" child. I went into her appointment the next day expecting that the biggest issue was whether or not she needed shots! When we arrived, they asked to update her family history. I thought I was prepared and quickly went through what I had done the day before with Rachel. But, after the nurse walked out I remembered that my mother-in-law has scoliosis. I thought nothing of it and almost didn't say anything, but thankfully I told the doctor shortly after he walked in. As he casually checked Katelyn's spine, he immediately saw there was a curve and said we needed to get an X-ray. The focus of the rest of the appointment was about her back. Everything else for a routine checkup was quickly forgotten.

Katelyn had no idea what was going on and her anxiety kicked in full force. The two of us headed to the X-ray room with the technician, where I was able to watch the images come up on the screen. Even without medical training, I could see her spine was curved! I didn't tell Katelyn, knowing that would cause even more anxiety.

Our doctor was wonderful with Katelyn. He took us back to the computer and showed us what appeared to be a small curve. He suggested we follow up with an orthopedic specialist, who would probably just monitor her curve every six months.

We left that day with a referral.

I don't know what her original Cobb angles were because he never told us and we didn't know to ask.

Truth be told, I knew very little about scoliosis. I remembered that a girl in my high school wore a very uncomfortable looking metal contraption because she had scoliosis, and that my mother-in-law had a spinal curvature that required surgery to have rods put in her back. I thought about how impossible it would be for Katelyn to wear a back brace to school. I didn't know what a Cobb angle was, and I didn't know there were different braces for different types of curves.

THE WAITING

A huge cloud was hanging over the start of seventh grade, as we waited to see the orthopedic doctor for Katelyn. Why does it take so long to get that first appointment? Sometimes I wish families in this situation were given priority because of the amount of emotional stress we are in.

To make matters worse, the orthopedist's office called a few days before her scheduled appointment to say that the doctor needed to take some time off and would have to reschedule our appointment. Now the wait was even longer! As I look back, I think it was only six weeks or so between her physical and the appointment with the surgeon, but it felt like forever! Unfortunately, the longer wait allowed us to do a lot more internet searching. What we found was a mix of helpful information and, of course, some scary information.

The appointment day finally arrived and I picked Katelyn up from school. It was a crazy experience. First, they took new X-rays. Then the doctor launched into a lengthy explanation of Katelyn's condition, most of which we didn't understand. What we heard was a distinctly mixed—and at times contradictory—message. The doctor told us that "nothing shows bracing works," and yet he went on to prescribe a brace. We were so confused. Why would a doctor tell us to do something that didn't work? He said bracing makes parents feel better—like they're doing something to have some control over the situation. Since I like feeling in control, bracing sounded good to me.

When we left the office, Katelyn was upset. I knew she would not be able to focus or learn the rest of the day, so we decided to stop by her school, collect her bag and tell them she would not be returning that day.

Exhausted and overwhelmed from all the information the orthopedic specialist threw at us, we now had to head straight to the orthotist.

The orthotist told us that Katelyn would be measured for a bending brace. Well, that didn't sound too bad, until he showed us an example. A bending brace doesn't mean you can bend in it, it means it bends you! And boy did it. One of the first mornings after sleeping in the brace, I asked Katelyn to bend over so I could check her back. Her curve was going in the other direction! What kind of a torture device does that? I resolved to keep my thoughts and opinions to myself and encouraged my daughter to have a positive attitude.

After many sleepless nights in the brace for Katelyn, the two of us headed back to the orthopedic doctor. He did not have a very good bedside manner and certainly didn't have a clue on how to talk with a preteen girl whose life had just been turned upside down. After that visit, I asked our general practitioner for a referral to someone else. On reflection, I should have done this sooner but I wanted to see if things would get better. I didn't think it was a lot to expect a doctor to have some compassion for his patients.

CHANGING DOCTORS

Changing physicians turned out to be the best decision we ever made. Our new referral took us two hours away to see orthopedic surgeon Dr. Stuart Weinstein. Our first appointment with Dr. Weinstein was amazing! He was well worth the drive, and even the subsequent long wait we had in his waiting room. Our spirits brightened when an amazing X-ray tech put Katelyn at ease and we felt reassured after our visit with Dr. Weinstein, who exuded a warm and comforting "everything-will-be-okay" attitude. We were so lucky to find him! It was kind of funny to learn that Dr. Weinstein published the BrAIST study proving that bracing was absolutely effective. It was quite a difference after hearing the first doctor say that all bracing did was make parents feel like they were doing something. I kind of wished I sent that doctor a copy of Dr. Weinstein's study, but I never did.

At the end of our first appointment, Dr. Weinstein recommended a new brace that Katelyn would need to wear 16 hours a day, rather than the bending brace that she only wore at night. Once I heard that I thought, "Uh oh...the girl who doesn't want anyone to know she has a brace is now supposed to wear this for 16 hours a day?" But, much to my surprise, Katelyn embraced the new brace and even started wearing it to school. She still hid it from friends and teachers but at least she was wearing it every day. It was another step in the right direction!

CURVY GIRLS

Even though Katelyn did everything that was asked of her, she clearly was not herself. Looking for answers on the internet I found a scoliosis support group, Curvy Girls, and that's when our lives completely changed. While on the Curvy Girls' website, I noticed information about their book, *Straight Talk with the Curvy Girls*. Knowing how much Katelyn loves to read, I thought it would be a good idea to buy her this book. Still, I hesitated because I had no idea what she would think of it. Up to that point she didn't want to talk about her scoliosis or have anyone mention anything about it. How would she react if I bought her a book all about scoliosis? Since her birthday was coming up, I decided to go ahead and order the book. The worst that could happen was that she would be angry at me. I also found a necklace to give to her that said, "Curvy Girl."

I don't remember how she reacted when she opened her birthday gifts. But I do remember that her attitude about scoliosis completely changed after reading the book and discovering that there were countless other girls out there who were going through pretty much the same thing that she was. Indeed, the book changed her so much that she wanted to start the first Iowa Curvy Girls' chapter.

Frankly, being a parent leader of a support group like that was not something that I felt I could do. "Let's just wait for someone else to start it," I said when Katelyn first broached the idea. Ironically, that was the beginning of Katelyn teaching me how to be strong and get out of my own comfort zone!

Within a few weeks of becoming the official Curvy Girls Iowa Leader, Katelyn and I began a new scoliosis chapter. This time we were a team. We weren't fighting and she was no longer angry at the world. That first meeting in October, we welcomed our first family into our heart and home.

Katelyn was very excited about her new role and took it upon herself to spread the word about the new chapter to as many girls as possible.

She convinced a local TV station to air a feature on Curvy Girls and did the interview in our home, speaking with confidence and never shying away from the camera. I watched from a distance, proud of my daughter's focus, determination, and sense of empowerment. She explained how she wanted to reach as many girls as possible to let them know that they were not alone. And that is exactly what she did!

Katelyn now owned her scoliosis story and shared it with anyone who would listen!

Why the complete change? Because of that book I bought her, *Straight Talk with the Curvy Girls*. By reading stories like this about other girls with scoliosis, she learned that she was not alone. She was not the only girl out there wearing a brace. And she was far from the only one experiencing those frightening visits with surgeons and orthotists. Instead, she learned there is a network of girls all over the world that have similar feelings.

It wasn't long after Katelyn started her group that we were attending our first Curvy Girls' convention. I was so nervous—certainly more nervous than my daughter was! I'm not very good with new people and I am very uncomfortable in unfamiliar situations. But with Katelyn by my side, I walked into the convention and met the most amazing women. Mothers and daughters had breakfast together that first morning, and then we went our separate ways; moms in one room and girls in another.

When we met for lunch a few hours later, we didn't even sit together! Mothers and daughters alike had established new relationships and bonded with others just like us. That's how comfortable each of us were with the new people we had just spent a very short amount of time with. The funniest thing was how Katelyn sat with the daughters of the moms I was sitting with! We learned so much about scoliosis and ourselves all within those couple of days at our first convention.

WHAT A DIFFERENCE A YEAR MAKES

The following August, Katelyn was entering the eigth grade. It was her back-to-school night and Katelyn decided to wear her brace on the outside of her clothes. Talk about change! This was a huge step from the girl who wanted to hide the brace and who would freak out if you mentioned the word scoliosis. I think for Katelyn, wearing the brace on the outside was a way for her to let her teachers know what was going on, without having to initiate the conversation. She might not have been ready to start a conversation about scoliosis, but she was ready and willing to answer their questions. What a difference a year makes. I was so proud of how far Katelyn had come.

After nearly three years of bracing, we were finally at Katelyn's last scoliosis appointment. As we sat in the waiting room, I saw a new family walk in. Suddenly, I was flooded with emotions and tears started running down my face. To this day I cannot explain why I had that reaction. I felt sadness, frustration, happiness, and fear in a matter of seconds. I think I felt all those emotions because I knew that the family sitting across from me had no idea what was ahead of them. I wanted to tell them not to worry about all the "what if's," and to urge them to take a deep breath, and just take it one day at a time. Everything would be okay.

When Katelyn was diagnosed with scoliosis, I thought back to the family history and wondered if she, too, would have to have the same kind of spinal fusion surgery that her grandmother had so many years ago. Would that be Katelyn's destiny as well? Those are the "what if's" we sometimes don't have control of. But what we do have control of is finding the right orthopedic surgeon and the right brace. We can all play an active role in our healthcare and push for the best treatment possible.

When your daughters are diagnosed with scoliosis and you see them sad and struggling, I hope you look to see if there is a local Curvy Girls' chapter near you. Having support is so important. For Katelyn, getting involved with Curvy Girls was a turning point. I think by leading her own group, helping girls feel less alone and scared, was also healing for her. While scoliosis might have changed her life at 13 years old, it also provided her with a new passion for helping others. Scoliosis is weird like that. It tests you greatly, but then gives us more than we expected in the end. For me, it brought Katelyn and I closer and showed me that my daughter was more resilient than I could have dreamed.

Today, Katelyn is an extremely confident, well-spoken young woman ready to conquer the world. And to think all the changes she made for herself started with a book!

Intisar

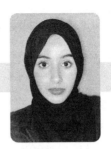

Meet Intisar from Kenya

Age: 23

Braced at 12

Spinal Surgery at age 14

Intisar likes to bake. She recently started an online baking business where she sells pastries and cakes. Intisar also loves to read and, on some days, enjoys binge watching Netflix

Being part of Curvy Girls gave Intisar the strength and confidence to be herself unapologetically. Blanketed in fear and shame, Intisar just wanted to be like everyone else her age.

Frustrated and desperate to find an effective treatment, this devoted mother-daughter team searched inside and outside of their country until they found a doctor they trusted.

Intisar's message: It gets easier. Time literally heals all wounds. I've been through a whole lot of hard days in my 23 years, but I have come out of each challenge victorious simply by believing and having faith that everything gets easier eventually. Also, surround yourself with powerful women. I had my mum, my sister, my boss, and Scolimama, Robin.

> **Intisar Mughal and her mum Shahida Mohamed**

Mama Has Your Back

THE DIAGNOSIS

Intisar: One morning while showering, I noticed my waist was indented more on one side compared to the other. I didn't think it was anything alarming, but I still told my mum.

Mum: At the time, she was only nine years old. I didn't think it was anything to worry about and so I told her to ignore it—it was just her waistline forming. And so she did.

Intisar: As a young girl, I remember always being the smallest and skinniest little human among my friends. I was also always tired. I remember when I was in the third grade, my school bag was huge and by the time I would carry it up the stairs to class, I was exhausted and needed a few minutes to catch my breath. But I still didn't think that was a real issue.

Mum: I did begin to notice that Intisar would get tired easily and that she wasn't standing straight. And when I saw her walk, it was beginning to look odd. I told her on various occasions to walk properly. At some point, I noticed she was standing weirdly with her legs crossed while she stood straight. "Intisar, why do you stand like that? Come here let me see what is happening."

Intisar: I couldn't stand straight. I had to lean on something all the time. One day my mum yelled furiously at me.

Mum: Out of my own frustration, I angrily asked her again, "What is wrong with you, Intisar? Stand straight and stop walking like that!"

Intisar: I had no explanation. I was confused. I thought I was standing straight. I would not do this purposely. I just felt comfortable standing and walking the way I did.

Mum: Now a bit more concerned, I immediately looked at her spine but was unable to see a problem. But nevertheless, I decided I would ask a doctor to look. A few days later, the doctor came to our home and I asked him to look at the way Intisar was walking and standing.

Intisar: The doctor asked me to walk back and forth. He concluded that my walking was a bit awkward. Then he told my mum that she should take me for an X-ray and then we will know.

And so it began. I recall that day vividly. I was dancing away at a school dance when my mum arrived. She said we have to go to the hospital and get that X-ray done.

Mum: Once the X-rays were completed, we got the results immediately. The radiologist was a young man who told me, "This is scoliosis and it has no other cure but surgery." I disregarded his comment and we went home as if it was like any other day. The results on the paper said she had idiopathic scoliosis. I stared at the diagnosis for a while trying to adjust to it. We then booked an appointment with an orthopedic surgeon from that exact hospital.

Intisar: I couldn't even pronounce it. Id-io-path-ic scoliosis? I was so confused. How could a spine grow like that?

Mum: I had no idea what to do with this information. What should we do or where do we go for help? No one in my family had any condition like this. Intisar is one of my four children and youngest of my two girls. We were normally healthy other than an occasional cold or at worst—food poisoning. But now they are telling us we need to see an orthopedic surgeon.

Intisar: I was terrified. At one point, my mum found me crying in the bathroom and asked me what was wrong. I told her that the spine is important and so since mine was "messed up," I would die.

Mum: Hearing the fear that my daughter was holding inside broke my heart. I immediately tried to console her, "No Intisar, don't say that, we will find a doctor and you will be healed. For now you will continue to be you and no one will ever know."

Intisar: By then, I had just started high school and was absolutely terrified that someone would find out that I had a crooked spine.

Mum: I must have taken Intisar to every single spine and bone doctor that there was in Kenya. Unfortunately, those visits did not go well. Each doctor gave us bad news or opinions that seemed uninformed.

OUR ENDLESS SEARCH FOR A DOCTOR

Intisar: Doctors have the ability to either break you or make you with their words. Every time we went to see another doctor, no treatment options were given. One particular doctor crudely pointed out that surgery was only required for cosmetic reasons and that I could live with the curves as it wouldn't affect my day-to-day life.

Mum: Living with an untreated case of scoliosis was not an option for my daughter. I was not going to watch my child go through the rest of her life slowly bending to one side. This is when I decided that our journey for help was not over; it was just beginning and I was more determined than ever to look for more doctors.

Intisar: My mum did what she had promised. She did not want to leave any professional out of the equation if they said they could help. But each of them was a disappointment.

Mum: One doctor we saw was a chiropractor with a very impressive looking office—along with a very pricey consultation fee. After he examined Intisar, he said if my daughter changed how she lived, and practiced his everyday exercises at home, along with a few physiotherapy sessions with him, her curve would move back to a straight spine. He asked her to carry a pillow with her everywhere she went and finally gave her an exercise tutorial print out.

Intisar: He cracked my bones and made me feel very relaxed. I even got a complementary massage. It was amazing. He told me I needed to get a stool and a pillow. I would carry the pillow around and place it every time I needed to sit so as to support my imbalanced body. The stool was to be kept at home when I needed to stand. He also gave me exercises to do every day and asked me to change my shoes. He said all these things would return my spine back to its normal curvature. I loved the visit for the massage but I knew there was no way a few changes in my life would return my 30° curve back to normal. My mum agreed with my sentiment, so we looked for yet another doctor.

SADDLES, CARDBOARD, AND MORE

Mum: Our journey to find answers continued. Off we drove 194.3 kilometers (about 120 miles), from Nairobi to Nanyuki to see some traveling doctors and hear what they had to say. They told us that there was a mission hospital, IAC Kijabe Hospital in Limuru, where we could get a scoliosis brace and everything would be good. And so we planned our trip to Limuru, which was about 70 kilometers from home.

Intisar: When we arrived at the hospital in Limuru, we saw a lovely doctor who told us bracing would halt the curvature. I was immediately taken in for sizing. I left there with this huge brown brace. And then I learned I had to wear it ALL DAY. I absolutely despised it and did not want it anywhere near me. One of my friends told me it looked like a horse's saddle. This was the beginning of a constant war between me and my mum.

Mum: Intisar was not happy at all when she saw this brace. But I am her mother and if they said the brace was going to stop her curve from progressing, then she had to wear this brace!

Every morning I would check to see if she had it on. And every morning there was a minor war, as Intisar would try to get out of wearing her brace. She absolutely hated wearing it.

Intisar: For the first month, I took it seriously and wore that saddle of a brace. Even though I would get overheated and have pain from wearing it, I kept it on. To make this more challenging, the brace was heavy—it weighed me down which made it difficult to walk. I felt like the brace was causing more problems on my already fragile body.

Going to school every day was a nightmare. The edges of the brace would literally pierce my flesh. Saying that I hated it was an understatement. Eventually, I got so sick of it that I just stopped wearing it.

Mum: As I continued to check her daily, it appeared she was still trying to run away from wearing the brace. What I didn't know was that sometimes she would have it on in the morning, go to school, and then remove it.

Intisar: I just didn't want it anymore. My friends in school made fun of me walking all around in the brace. They didn't understand that by wearing the brace it held my spine from progressing. My so-called friends continued to mock me every day, laughing, saying I was "plastic." They would just call my brace the "Horse thing." I was now becoming emotionally sick from it and just told my mum I don't want it, and will NOT wear it anymore!

Mum: A big part of me understood why Intisar felt this way but I still wanted her to wear her brace. I needed to buy more time to find another solution. As a parent, I realized that her refusal to wear the brace all day would only allow her scoliosis to get worse. I felt like I was running out of time.

Intisar: That year we travelled to the coast for holiday. The temperature would get up to 40°C (104°F), so I completely gave up. I just couldn't wear it any longer—being in that heat is what made me completely stop. And yes, my choice to stop wearing the brace had a huge impact on what the next X-ray revealed. My curve was progressing and my hate for the brace was too. They were directly proportional. The new X-rays revealed that bracing was no longer an option.

Mum: I think I was in denial. I truly didn't think it would come to this. All I saw when I looked at my daughter was someone healthy. But the reality was that her body was changing. I could already see how much she was bending to one side. I didn't want her to have surgery and I didn't want this to get any worse. I kept my fears to myself and it was silently killing me how quickly everything was happening.

Intisar: We saw another surgeon and he said surgery was the only solution left. But he said we could never do the complex procedure in Kenya because it would not be successful and consequences would lead to paralysis.

Mum: I could not even begin to process what we heard. I became more determined in my search for hospitals that could perform this type of surgery—or at least offer us another solution.

Intisar: I wanted life to go back to normal. I just wanted to go back to school and forget all about this. But my mum does not give up that easily. And this is where we hit rock bottom and met one of the most bizarre healers in all of the years of my life. He was the "let's straighten her with cardboard and elastoplasts/Band Aids™" healer.

Mum: This healer or masseur was a traditional Indian doctor and he had this brilliant idea that Intisar's spine could be straightened using elastoplast. Yes, the gauze you use when you have a cut. He literally pasted it all over her back and told me to return after a few weeks. And of course, he charged us an enormous amount of money. But I was desperate, so we did it.

Intisar: That night, I did not sleep at all. I woke the whole house up because I was itchy, irritable, and frustrated. I woke my sister up and had her literally blowing into it and rubbing it, trying to help me sleep. Nothing. The next day, I had to go to school and was not comfortable at all. My back was so irritated. On the second day, I came home and after my shower it started coming off and so water was getting inside which made it slowly begin to peel off.

We returned to his office and not thinking matters could get any worse, he surprised us even more. He literally took cardboard and stuck it to my back. My mum looked at him. Laughed, and removed it all. That was the end of me being pasted.

THE PROMISE

Mum: One day while reading the newspaper, I read about a surgeon who might be able to help us. At this point we had seen so many doctors that we were both emotionally exhausted. It was unfortunate that after all this time we still hadn't found anyone we liked even a little. But I was trying to remain optimistic, so I made an appointment with this new surgeon. We were both happily surprised.

Intisar: This is the doctor that won me over. He was different. He told me that spinal fusion surgery was our next stop and that he would personally perform it. He looked at my mum and me that day, and promised us that I would come out of it perfectly okay. He said surgery was essential and time was of the essence.

Mum: We finally had a surgeon we liked and trusted. Finally! Our next mission was raising funds for an immediate surgery and Alhamdulillah (praise to God) we raised it. I did all that I could to make this happen but we could have never done this without the generosity of so many of our friends, as well as anonymous donors. It was because of these people that Intisar was able to have this surgery. I will be forever grateful. Raising money for an impromptu surgery is definitely not a joke. Not every family member took Intisar being operated on as well as I expected. However, I had to be strong for my daughter. So, I put on my big girl shoes and knew what I had to do.

Intisar: I recalled one specific person's generosity—who until today has remained anonymous. He called my mum and told her he would pay for our flight to India where the doctors would perform the surgery. We were so grateful and asked why. He said his wife had been in a wheelchair due to spine issues and this was the least he could do. It was so touching because he knew nothing about me other than that I needed to have this surgery.

Mum: The whole process of raising funds was very stressful and emotional for me. All I knew was that I had to do whatever it would take for Intisar to have this operation. It all seemed so surreal, but we finally had all the money and were on our way.

Intisar: After a long flight, we arrived in India at 3 a.m. It felt like a dream. When we landed, we were told to go straight to the hospital and were given a room to sleep. The next day, I was scheduled for many pre-operative tests—X-rays, MRIs and blood tests.

Mum: At this point, no date was given when the surgery would actually take place. We were told it could be the following day or a week. Not knowing just made things a little more intense.

Intisar: The day of my surgery came with no warning. It was 5am and I was awakened abruptly by two nurses in a frenzy. While half asleep, they were both trying to change my clothing into scrubs, plate my hair, and remove my earrings. I was scared, tired and just wanted to be left alone but that was not going to happen.

Mum: We did not know surgery was to happen on that day; they caught us by surprise. I could not understand why they were rushing. I was still trying to wake up and process what was going on when they handed me Intisar's personal belongings while pushing her bed out the door. I tried to quickly dress and follow but they were gone. I stood outside the doors of the operating rooms hoping they would let me in but I was not allowed. I just wanted to say goodbye and tell her not to worry but that never happened.

TIME FOR SURGERY, TIME FOR PRAYER

Intisar: As I was being rolled into the operating theater, it became very real—surgery was happening. I began to pray. I kept asking for my mum but she wasn't allowed in. I remember being upset because the IV that they had placed in my wrist hurt. I was also very cold. I looked around the room and just started to cry. My surgeon saw how scared I was and immediately stopped and sat down next to me. He got me a heater and massaged my wrist where the IV was put in.

I felt lucky to have a very compassionate and kind person for a surgeon. He once again looked at me and said, "I promise you, you will be okay." I think I needed to hear that. I believed him and began to feel a little better.

Mum: Even though I knew Intisar was in good hands, I was still very nervous. Once I was informed that the surgery was beginning, I broke down. I think I needed a quiet moment alone to release all my built-up fears; I never wanted Intisar to see me this scared. I tried to get my mind off the surgery, so I left the hospital to buy all her favorite food and snacks for when she woke up.

They told me the surgery should take six to eight hours. When the time had passed, panic began to set in. To help me cope with the added hours of waiting, I called home and told the family what was happening. My children assured me they were all praying and would not stop until they heard their sister was out of surgery. Nearly fourteen hours later, the surgeon finally came out. I, unfortunately, never asked what took so long. I was just happy to learn she was alive and doing well.

Intisar: The first person I saw when I began to wake was my mum. She was crying and smiling. I asked her why she was crying but I don't remember what she said. I also remember the doctor being there asking me to move my legs. I did and then fell back to sleep.

Mum: As a parent, we cannot truly relax until the surgery is actually over and you're standing next to your daughter holding her hand. Once

Intisar was awake, I never wanted to leave her side. They took her to ICU. Her face was swollen from surgery and she looked so pale. I was amazed at the fact that they had her lying on her back after this surgery. When speaking with the surgeon, he said the fusion was a success and Intisar would make a full recovery.

Intisar: My experience during surgery is like a dream. It happened so fast. I felt like my doctors knew me personally and that they were honestly the best doctors anyone could ask for. They did an incredible job of taking care of me. My scar isn't the same as other scoliosis surgery scars, as it is located on my side. The doctors believed having the scar on the side of my body would be easier to conceal, than having it on my back. He told me he wanted me to always feel confident.

Mum: They kept Intisar in the ICU for three or four days and then brought her to a regular ward where she spent another 10 days. To continue her recovery, we stayed at a guesthouse near the hospital for another month and a half. When she needed to see her surgeon for checkups, she was taken by ambulance. I was so appreciative and thankful for the care that Intisar was given.

The kindness of others continued as we began to plan our trip back home. To ensure our flight back to Kenya did not cause any problems, the airline made sure she had a very comfortable seat. Everything was going as well as our surgeon had promised.

RECOVERY

Intisar: What my mum did for me during my long recovery is something that I will never forget or be able to repay. She fed me and bathed me. She sat with me when I could not sleep and encouraged me to always pray. Then there were the million small things she did like buying all my favorite snacks, and constantly paying for additional time on my phone so I could talk to my friends back in Kenya. She went above and beyond to try and make my experience as tolerable as possible. I've thanked her so many times but those two little words just aren't enough to convey my appreciation for everything she did and sacrificed for me. She is the strongest person in my scoliosis journey and I will forever consider her the real hero of my story.

Mum: I don't look at myself as a hero—a mother, yes, but not a hero. We all do what we need to for our children. Making sure Intisar had the best surgeon and care was my number one priority. No one wants to put their child through this procedure and not have her return home better than she left. Were there many challenges? Yes. But at the end, you want to know it was all worth it.

Intisar: During my recovery at home my life slowly picked up right where it left off. All my friends came to see me; some came every day. We would binge watch shows and eat snacks. My family spoiled me by never allowing me to do anything. My mum made sure my room was stocked with everything I could possibly need.

After three months of staying home, I was ready to go back to school. I rarely talked about my scoliosis or the surgery. Not talking about it was easy for me, however, it was never completely out of my mind. The scar across my torso was a constant reminder. My doctors offered to have my scar changed with plastic surgery, but I refused. Over time I learned to love it and accept it. I am a true believer that the first step in healing from this type of surgery is to love yourself unconditionally. But this was something easier said than done. I knew what I needed to do to make a full physical recovery. I needed to put in the work and get myself just as strong on the inside.

HEALING FROM WITHIN

Trying to reflect on different forms of self-love, I would often scroll through my phone. Like most girls my age, I live on all forms of social media. On this one day as I was scrolling on Instagram, I found a post by the American celebrity, Kylie Jenner. Kylie had reposted a picture of a teenage ballerina with scoliosis and tagged Curvy Girls Scoliosis. Fascinated by the beautiful photo, I was also intrigued to learn more about this group and decided to Google them.

Once on the Curvy Girls' website, something inside me wanted to know more. I immediately emailed Robin Stoltz, the founder's mom, to ask additional questions.

Reaching out to Robin was the best thing I have ever done. I would soon learn that Robin was the most understanding person I had ever spoken to. She was so kind and lovely. The more she told me about Curvy

Girls, the more excited I became. My mum and I always talked about beginning something in Kenya that would help families who were going through similar struggles—and it finally looked like it could be possible. Robin was like my little fairy Godmother, as she helped us make one of our dreams become a reality.

A few months later, I became the official Curvy Girls International Leader of Kenya.

Mum: When Intisar first told me about this support group, I was confused. I never heard of this kind of support for scoliosis. But seeing her so motivated and excited made me want to help as well. Who better than me can know the fears of hearing the words idiopathic scoliosis and surgery for the first time? If I could help other parents not make the mistakes we went through, then my experiences with Intisar would have been all worth it.

Intisar: As a new leader there was so much to learn. Luckily for me, Robin told me that Curvy Girls was hosting their third international conference that year. All new leaders needed to arrive a day in advance so they could be trained on how to run a chapter—learn how to find members and actually run activities. I wanted to go and so did my mum but traveling across the world for two people was very expensive. We did our best to try and raise money but it was not enough. That's when we learned that the Curvy Girls Foundation found someone to sponsor our trip. My mum and I were very excited and honored that they were able to make this happen for us.

Arriving at the hotel felt surreal. I couldn't believe I was here—in New York attending my first convention. Meeting all the girls with scoliosis gave me a serious confidence boost, especially seeing with my own eyes that I was not the only one with scoliosis. It was such a wonderful experience but it was definitely a culture shock. The American lifestyle is very different from the Kenyan lifestyle.

Mum: I didn't know what to expect coming to this convention especially with it being Ramadhan, but I was very happy we went. It was wonderful to talk to the other parents. I began to worry less about Intisar for the first time after attending the conference. For so long, I worried if she would be able to just be a typical girl after her surgery. I was so relieved to see that so many girls who had surgery were happy while continuing to do what they wanted. This conference brought me genuine relief as I watched my daughter jumping around, laughing, and dancing with the other girls. I was finally reassured that she too would be okay.

Intisar: Being at the convention, I realized how lucky I was. My experience with scoliosis was pretty hard at the start, and surgery was tough. Still today I can only see the positive effects it has had on me. It made me stronger and transformed me into a resilient young woman. I thank God every day that my scoliosis journey led me to such beautiful, kind people who taught me to love myself.

FINAL THOUGHTS

Intisar: Now that my scoliosis treatment is over, I often think if I was given a wish to be able to go back in time and give one piece of advice to my younger-self, what would it be?

I would tell that girl to be kinder to herself. This thing called scoliosis is not that scary. You might think it's going to destroy you or ruin your life, but it's not. Instead, you will one day be empowered to help other girls feel less afraid. You will become part of a peer led support system that is helping to remove the stigma that comes with this condition. So dry your tears and take a deep breath. You will accomplish more than you ever thought. The best is yet to come.

It took a Curvy Girls' convention and meeting so many girls who are so proud of saying those words to get me to finally accept it and say it out loud, without tearing up or lying about it. My name is Intisar Mughal and I have scoliosis.

WHERE INTISAR IS TODAY

Today, Intisar continues to raise scoliosis awareness in her country, while growing her Curvy Girls' group and helping other girls through treatment, She recently completed her undergraduate law program and plans to practice law in the future.

Sophie

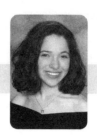

Meet Sophie from New York

Age: 15

Braced at 14

Actively doing the Schroth Method

Sophie enjoys teaching ukulele on the weekends and participating in the marching band and wind ensemble at high school.

Sophie has shared that Curvy Girls has helped her immensely throughout her scoliosis diagnosis and treatment by offering guidance, advice, and support.

Sophie was determined to not allow a back brace or the curve in her spine to define her. Armed with information, Sophie found herself combatting her scoliosis with grace and perseverance.

Personal Message: It's easier to go through this journey when you have friends to lean on.

Part 1: Memoirs

Sophie Klein and her mother Cara Harth

The Strength Within

Sophie

"You never know how strong you are, until being strong is your only choice."
—Bob Marley

I had just turned 14 when I was diagnosed with scoliosis. It was October and I was at my yearly check-up when my pediatrician asked me to lean forward for the Adams Forward Bend test, a pretty typical routine for as long as I can remember. I remember reassuring myself, "This won't last long. I'll stand up in two seconds. Things like this don't happen to me." Little did I know how wrong I was.

The doctor called my mom into the room and said, "It looks like Sophie might have a very minor degree of rotation, maybe 5°." He advised Mom to double check with an orthopedic specialist. Mom seemed worried; me, not so much. After all, I heard the doctor say "minor" curve, so how bad could it be? I doubted that I had scoliosis. That would be crazy.

When I got home, I texted my best friends to tell them that the doctor thought I had a minor curve in my back. One of my best friends who has scoliosis had to have spinal fusion surgery three years earlier, so this wasn't terribly unfamiliar territory for me.

A couple of days later, my dad picked me up after school to take me for X-rays and to meet with the orthopedist. While I was being X-rayed, my dad stayed in the booth with the technician. When my film images came up on the screen, I heard my dad exclaim, "That's her?"

"This can't be good," I thought to myself. There was apparently a very clear "S" shape to my spine that none of us had expected. It was so pronounced that my dad, with no radiology training, could recognize it. We went to the exam room and waited for the orthopedist. I told my dad that I hoped I didn't have to wear a brace because that would be terrible. Have you seen the brace they make you wear for scoliosis? I'm not going to lie. At first glance, it looks pretty scary. It's the shape of a person's torso, but a bit bent out of shape.

Dr. C. came in quickly and prescribed a Boston brace. At first I was upset but then I realized even though a brace wasn't ideal, it was better than having no options and going straight to surgery. I left that day feeling that we had a solid treatment plan; however, after we got home my parents seemed to be thinking differently. My dad ended the day clearly fearful of the journey that was ahead and how it would affect me. I was actually pretty relaxed about the whole thing, probably because I didn't have a clue about the impact a scoliosis diagnosis could have. Shortly after getting home, my parents were on the internet reading about other types of scoliosis treatments. That's when they decided to take me for a second opinion.

Meanwhile, my older brother emailed me a link for Curvy Girls, a teen-run scoliosis support group, and reminded me that he had seen flyers posted all around our school. They were everywhere—the hallways, bathrooms, gym, nurse's office, and even outside the cafeteria. He suggested that I look into it and attend a meeting. I would later learn that Val, who also has scoliosis, put the flyers up to help other girls who were newly diagnosed realize they did not have to be alone.

FINDING A DOCTOR & A BRACE

I reached out to my best friend Katya who had had scoliosis surgery. Later that night, her mom called to offer my mom some advice. She told us about Dr. Michael Vitale at Columbia Children's Hospital where she'd taken her daughter. A few days later, my parents and I took a day off from school and work and went to see Dr. Vitale. I was a bit more nervous about this visit because not only was it at a hospital, but it was in New York City. For some reason, going into the city makes me nervous.

This visit was a completely different experience. Dr. Vitale measured my two curves, which were both 28°. He talked to us about Schroth physical therapy, 3D bracing, the benefits of taking vitamin D supplements, and handed us a flyer for Curvy Girls.

After meeting with the doctor, we went down the hall and met with John from East Coast Orthotics, who took scans to make my Rigo brace. After John was finished with all the measurements, he asked me to pick a color or design pattern for my brace. Initially, I wanted only white, thinking that would be the best option for all my clothes. That was until I caught sight of a pink brace sticking out of a cabinet. When I saw the pink, I immediately fell in love with it and that's when I decided to change from white to pink. John also gave us a Curvy Girls' flyer, which just helped confirm that it would be beneficial for all of us to attend.

After the visit at Columbia, my parents may have been overwhelmed but at least we left feeling much more informed and prepared for the journey that lay ahead. Over the next couple of weeks, while waiting for my brace to be made, I began taking vitamin D and made contact with Curvy Girls. And what luck, the original chapter was only one town away. A few days after we saw Dr. Vitale, my parents and I attended our first Curvy Girls' support group.

GIRLS LIKE ME!

I remember the anticipation of that first meeting. I hadn't gotten my brace yet and was still adjusting to the whole idea of having scoliosis. Everything was so unfamiliar; it all seemed so strange. A whole group of people with scoliosis like me? I didn't know what to expect.

I actually thought it was going to be a serious kind of meeting but it was nothing like I thought. When I got there, I was relieved to see a group of smiling girls just like me. My first meeting was wonderful. They answered all of my questions about bracing. We also shared a lot of laughs as they told funny stories about their braces, and talked about how having scoliosis doesn't have to be a bad thing. Since that first meeting, I've gone to every meeting I could. I had no idea how much Curvy Girls would become such an influential part of my scoliosis journey.

THE BRACE ARRIVES

It was over Thanksgiving break when we picked up my brace. When John came into the room, he was holding my pink brace. It was actually kind of pretty, considering it was a scoliosis brace. He helped me put it on for the first time. I wasn't at all sure what it was going to feel like. It certainly didn't feel natural to be wearing something like that. John kindly went over how to put the brace on and showed me how tight it ultimately needed to be worn. While it wasn't comfortable, I felt confident that I could adjust to wearing it. My goal was to work myself up to wearing this for 22 hours a day. John suggested that I first get used to sleeping in my brace and then once I could make it through the night, to start wearing it in the afternoon. About two weeks later, I was ready to take the next step—wearing the brace to school. It's better not to keep your brace a secret. When you're ready, you should tell your peers.

I remembered we talked about this idea during one of my first Curvy Girls' meetings. In the back of my mind, I knew it was great advice but at the same time I wasn't ready to take that step, not just yet. It took me a while to feel comfortable telling all my friends about my brace and diagnosis, but eventually I did. I didn't want to deal with the stress of a secret, but I also didn't want to be seen as "the girl with scoliosis."

While first wearing my brace, I was supercautious, always pulling my shirt down in the back. God forbid a kid saw my brace peeking out during class or in the hallway. From the beginning, I was able to tell my two best friends about it because I trusted that they would be there to support me. And if they weren't, I honestly would have been dodging a bullet because that would have only shown me that they weren't true friends. That being said, I debated whether to tell the rest of my friend group. Once I did, I felt so much better because I was no longer keeping that difficult secret inside.

A few months later, while sitting in class my teacher asked students to talk about "objects that were important to them." After giving it some thought, I decided to talk about my back brace and raised my hand to speak. I was really nervous to share because I hadn't spoken about it in this class, but it was also very liberating to talk about it with everyone. That moment in class empowered me to feel more confident. Surprisingly, some of my friends actually found it pretty cool.

I think this was one of my first turning points with scoliosis because I slowly stopped caring if people saw my brace at school. If my shirt was stuck up in the back, I might be embarrassed for a second but I learned to just laugh at myself and move on. It took me a while but I had to realize for myself that my brace was nothing to be embarrassed of. There's absolutely nothing wrong with wearing a back brace! Everyone has to sit up straight all day; we curvy girls could just use a bit more help. I'm grateful to my brace for physically supporting me all that time. In the morning while dressing for school, I sometimes used to imagine that I was a superhero, maybe a scoliosis superhero, and that my brace was my armor. With my brace, nothing could get in my way and I was sort of invincible.

Eventually, I decided to tell the rest of my friends about my brace. Once I did, I noticed something. The more comfortable I felt, the more open they were to talk to me about my brace. Mentioning an upcoming doctor appointment, or that I had to go to the nurse to take off my brace before I could meet them at lunch, actually encouraged them to ask questions. It also showed that I wasn't embarrassed. The key is to do it casually and it should work out great.

MARGUERITE

As I continued to deal with this new and unfamiliar condition, I began to notice that my family wasn't really sure how to talk about my diagnosis and brace, especially at family events like Thanksgiving. It almost seemed awkward. For months, my parents referred to my brace as, "the brace" instead of "your brace," which bothered me because it made it feel like more of a scary medical device, rather than something that had become very close and important to me. I shared how I was feeling about this with my mom. After reading Rachel's story in the first edition of *Straight Talk with the Curvy Girls*, my mom suggested that we name my brace, just as Rachel had done, in order to normalize talking about it. I liked that idea because it reinforced positive thoughts about my brace. After a few minutes of discussion, we collectively decided to name her "Marguerite." She was named after a butterfly in a children's book that I once treasured. It was almost as if I was a caterpillar carefully being protected and allowed to mature inside my own cocoon. Soon I would emerge from my cocoon, Marguerite, as a graceful butterfly.

MY OWN PERSONAL SCHROTH STUDIO

In early January, my dad and I headed back into the city for my first in-brace X-rays. X-rays taken of my spine while braced would tell us if the brace was effectively holding my curves from progressing. After the images were taken, we waited in the exam room for the results. When Dr. Vitale came in and pulled up my X-rays on his screen, he had good news. My in-brace curve degrees measured 5 and 9! The brace was absolutely working.

After several months of wearing my brace, I finally had my first appointment to learn scoliosis-specific exercises called the Schroth Method. I started in early January but the timing was not the greatest. It was right around midterms week at school and I was also starting daily rehearsals for my school play. I already had a lot on my plate, so adding in my scoliosis exercises was very overwhelming. One of the first things I quickly learned is that there is a tremendous amount of information to process, which included being aware of my body in a way I never had before. In order to learn this concept well, I had to see my Schroth physical therapist, Jeanann, twice a week during this very busy time of the school year.

In order to make this work, I prioritized my PT appointments around my other responsibilities. For instance, I skipped the school show rehearsal on Tuesday nights and drove one hour each way to see Jeanann. This did not include the additional practice time I needed to do at home. The only solution I could come up with was waking up half an hour earlier, so that I could do my exercises in the morning instead of after school when I had homework or stayed late for extra help. Initially, this new routine was challenging but it was what worked best for me. To ensure I had every opportunity to receive the best outcome, my parents installed a wall board with bars and some mirrors in my basement so I could do my exercises the same way I was doing with Jeanann. We bought a yoga mat and other pieces of equipment like poles and a yoga ball. For motivation, I listened to my favorite playlist and hung up an inspirational poster on the mirror. I call this area of the basement my "Schroth Studio."

Recently, when I was having trouble finding motivation to do my Schroth, Rachel gave me some great advice. She explained that when she was in the same situation, she thought about how she had no control over anything that was happening with her scoliosis, but something that she DID have control over was Schroth. After she said that, I began to think about when my parents and orthotist put me in a brace. It was something I was told to do. But the Schroth Method was something that I had control of, something I could do all on my own. At times it was intimidating, but it was also empowering to think how I was helping myself a great deal just by being in my Schroth studio exercising every morning. I also started doing a one-minute meditation after every workout. It not only serves as motivation to exercise for the full 30 minutes, but it helps me relax and reflect afterwards. Now I enjoy going down to my Schroth studio because it's serene and calm, and I am in control.

I still struggle sometimes to do my exercises daily and find motivation. What I've learned through this process is that Schroth is a gradual skill that is mastered over months, maybe years. It is a slow process but one of the perks of having scoliosis is that it builds resilience and patience. All I can do is put in the effort and the time because at the end of the day I will master it!

THE PAYOFF

My first out-of-brace X-ray was in August. It was the day after I came home from sleepaway camp. I felt very anxious leading up to this visit. This X-ray would show the degrees of my angles without the support of my brace. It would also confirm if the Schroth exercises were effective.

When it was time for the images to be taken, I made sure to stand up straight. While waiting for the technician to give me the next instruction, a crazy thought popped into my head, "What would happen if there was no improvement? What if my curves were worse?" All these "what ifs" started to occupy my thinking.

When we joined Dr. Vitale in the exam room, my heart felt like it was beating a little faster waiting for my image to appear on the screen. When I finally saw my X-ray, I couldn't believe it was me. My spine looked so straight! Dr. Vitale measured my angles to at 9° and 16°. My dad jumped up and started dancing in the middle of the room. I was ecstatic!

All of my efforts were paying off. Wearing my brace 22 hours a day and waking up early to exercise was all worth it. That was by far one of my favorite days because it was then that we realized that bracing was working and I would not need to worry about having surgery. We all finally saw the light at the end of the tunnel. I was instructed to keep wearing my brace and continue to exercise, with the hope of weaning in December.

Four months later, my next out-of-brace X-rays were scheduled. In order to get a more accurate representation of my curves, I would be out of my brace for 48 hours. In addition to the usual X-rays of my spine, a hand X-ray was ordered to determine how much growth I had remaining. After one year of wearing my brace and nearly 11 months of consistently working hard doing my Schroth exercises, I waited anxiously for the results.

When Dr. Vitale walked in the room, I kind of knew from the smile on his face that the results were good. My new Cobb degrees both measured 16°. A big difference from the original measurements of 28 and 28! My good news continued when the hand X-rays verified that I was completely done growing and I was officially ready to start weaning out of my brace!

Ironically, as happy as I was to receive such great news, I also had a small amount of guilt. Being around so many other girls with scoliosis, I realize that some patients could do everything right and yet still not have this outcome. Even now that I'm towards the end of my journey, I feel like I got off easy. I was diagnosed, did Schroth, wore a three-dimensional brace for a little over a year and saw great improvements. My curve degrees reversed and now I can start weaning. I feel so fortunate to have had this outcome.

I am weaning out of my brace at a rate of one hour per week. Most girls are excited when they find out they are getting out of their brace, but I have mixed feelings. Much to the surprise of a lot of people, I actually love my brace. It helped me. It stopped my curves from progressing and it helped with my back pain. For this reason, I was afraid that I would have a hard time weaning because I know physically and emotionally how much Marguerite has done for me. Although it has been a transition, I'm slowly trying to get used to not having her daily support. Ironically, I also just got my orthodontic braces off, so my family jokes that I got all of my braces off at the same time. I always thought it was funny how I used to get light pink bands on my orthodontic braces to match my back brace. It was part of embracing my brace instead of being ashamed of it.

GIVING BACK

Now that I'm nearing the end of my journey with scoliosis, I have had some time to look back and reflect on the obstacles that have been thrown at me during this past year. There is a Bob Marley quote that resonates with me as it helps me find inspiration from all that I've been through. "You never know how strong you are, until being strong is your only choice."

I feel like I was thrown into this adversity because I'm strong enough to live it, and I've come out on the other side of this even stronger. Of course, nobody wants scoliosis. I wouldn't say that I'm happy to have scoliosis, but what I've learned from my experience I wouldn't trade for anything. At one time or another, everybody faces challenges in their lives—and for us curvy girls, scoliosis *is* our challenge. It's our moment to prove our strength not just to the world, but to ourselves.

Never underestimate your own determination and strength. After having gone through scoliosis, I know that I can do anything. No matter what happens, whether you have a fairly simple journey like I did or if you need surgery, you too will be okay on the other side. Even though it may look dark, frightening, and intimidating now, there is a light shining at the end of your tunnel too. A light brighter than you could have ever imagined.

Today, I am proud and excited that my next stage in my scoliosis journey is to give back what I was so lucky to have received by accepting the position as the next Curvy Girls' coleader of the original Long Island group. My goal is to have new families feel as welcome and comfortable as my family did when we attended our very first Curvy Girls' meeting.

WHERE SOPHIE IS TODAY

Sophie no longer wears a brace but continues in her commitment to her Schroth routine. Creativity and enthusiasm, coupled with a strong desire to motivate and support other young girls led to her role as coleader for Curvy Girls of Long Island. Sophie plans to attend college to major in Neuroscience on a pre-med track towards a career in medicine.

Guilt, Anxiety & Resilience

Cara

My experience of Sophie's scoliosis diagnosis started out with a tremendous amount of guilt, overwhelming sadness, and anxiety. Fortunately, things improved.

At Sophie's annual checkup, shortly after she turned 14, the pediatrician mentioned she thought there was a small amount of scoliosis. I downplayed this and was dismissive, thinking tons of people have minor amounts of scoliosis and there was no urgency to deal with this. However, my *hypochondriacal* worrying husband wanted her to see an orthopedist ASAP. We were able to get Sophie in to see an orthopedist one week later. I couldn't get out of work that day so my husband took her. He texted me a picture of her X-ray from the office.

What I saw in the image left me stunned. My beautiful, intelligent, amazing, perfect daughter had a spine that looked like an "S." There was no doubt that she had scoliosis, and it was more serious than the pediatrician had suggested. The guilt hit me like a ton of bricks. A mix of guilt, overwhelming sadness, and anxiety washed over me—and I struggled to keep my emotions in check.

How did I not see this on her? I was the mother who exclusively breastfed, who fed her family organic food, who used only "natural" household cleaners. How was I not paying attention enough to notice the curvature in my daughter's spine? How could I not be there for her when she received the diagnosis?

When my husband texted me that image of Sophie's spine, he wrote that he felt sick to his stomach just looking at her X-ray. His reaction was one of shock, but the truth was that neither of us had expected the diagnosis. I was still at work and only starting to process the information. I just reassured him that we'd get through it, not really considering what it all meant.

Fortunately, the orthopedist spent a lot of time with them during that initial visit, measuring her angles and offering his recommendation for a Boston brace. There was no discussion of specific types of brace or any additional treatments that may be needed. He assured Sophie that she wouldn't be in the brace forever and that he would not send her to college with the brace.

TEARS, WORRY, AND THE UNKNOWN

We went to the orthotist shortly thereafter. He was nice enough, measured Sophie, and gave her the opportunity to ask a ton of questions. Unfortunately, none of us knew the right questions to ask.

The next few days and weeks were filled with lots of angst and tears for the family. Whenever I was alone I burst into tears. It's hard to drive a car when you're crying. My husband said he wished he could have the scoliosis instead of her. I was never truly worried about the scoliosis itself or needing surgery. Maybe that was ignorant but I just wasn't worried about that aspect of the diagnosis. Mostly I was worried about Sophie's self-esteem. Here she was on the cusp of adolescence, establishing her self-esteem, learning about her body and body image, developing her own style, fashion sense, and sense of self. She was starting to "look" at boys. And now she was going to be thrown into a brace that distorted all of that—or so I thought.

As much as we tried to shield Sophie from our own anxiety and worry, Sophie could sense it. She also knew that one of our big fears was how she would handle everything. I remember Sophie saying in the car that of all the things my husband and I had to worry about, one thing she did not want us to worry about was how she was handling everything. She insisted she was fine. That helped a tremendous amount. And ultimately, she was right. Of all the things we had to deal with on this journey, she always dealt with it like a champ.

DOING OUR HOMEWORK

Soon after she was measured for the Boston brace, we started doing our homework. We started reading articles, research papers, and talking to other parents of kids with scoliosis. That's when we realized there were other types of braces, and there was this mysterious thing called Schroth therapy. And we learned that the first physician you see is not always the physician who has all the answers. This was another one of those guilty moments. Why did we not do our homework earlier? Why were we not more informed? Why didn't we question the physician at all?

Guilt. What about my son? Was he not upset that Sophie's scoliosis completely monopolized our thoughts? Did he not feel jealous? Apparently, he was not. I asked him. Somehow, throughout this journey, my children have been the strongest members of this family. He completely supported everything that his sister and parents were going through. He was ready to put his own issues on the back burner whenever we needed him to do so.

On the advice of a dear friend, we ended up getting a second opinion. Sophie's best friend had scoliosis a few years earlier. I spoke to her mother who insisted that we get a second opinion in Manhattan. She also educated me about the Rigo brace (while my husband was simultaneously pouring over information online), and about this crazy therapy called the Schroth Method. It really did sound crazy, but perhaps it was something that we should explore.

By the time we had our appointment with the second orthopedist a few weeks later, we were already confident that we needed a Rigo-type brace and Schroth therapy. Sophie's angles were measured as thoracic 28° and lumbar 28°. The new orthopedist agreed with the need for a Rigo brace and Schroth, and also told Sophie that she needed to take more vitamin D. Even the number of hours of brace wearing that he recommended was higher than the recommendation of the first orthopedist. It was also remarkable how he treated Sophie like an adult. The orthopedist didn't just talk to my husband and me, but spoke directly to Sophie. He made sure that *she* understood what was going on.

VISITING A MULTI-DISCIPLINARY OFFICE

The entire multi-disciplinary operation at the new orthopedist's office was completely different, and even included low-radiation X-ray equipment and an on-site orthotist to measure Sophie for the new brace immediately. The orthotist was incredible, and spent a ton of time with us and with Sophie. He also made sure to talk to Sophie just as much, if not more, than he spoke to us. And of course, both the orthopedist and the orthotist recommended our angel of a Schroth therapist, Jeanann McGuffin. Later, we would learn that the orthotist would be working hand-in-hand with our Schroth therapist to achieve the best outcome for Sophie. The two of them would often confer about her brace and her X-rays.

Before Sophie actually started Schroth therapy, she had an initial 90-minute evaluation from the therapist. I have never seen anyone do an evaluation like this before. Jeanann has magic eyes and magic hands. She saw things in Sophie I just could not see. She immediately noticed her flat, pronated feet, and suggested she get foot orthotics to assist with keeping everything straight, from top to bottom. She would get down on the floor with Sophie to show her exercises. She has an incredible talent for teaching teenage girls about their own bodies, their own spines, their own curves, and making sure these kids truly understand how to make their own spinal corrections. Jeanann is not only a Schroth therapist, but also a listener, cheerleader, supporter, and motivator.

MAKING IT ALL WORK

We built Sophie a "Schroth studio" in our house. She has a private space in the basement with Schroth bars, mirrors, and music. It was never hard to get Sophie to want to do her exercises, what was hard was finding the time. She already had high demands on her schedule because of her high school workload. The Schroth therapy necessitated more time still, and the best way to fit that in was at home. For Sophie and her brother, high school started very early in the morning, and there was always a lot of drama finding time to fit everything into her daily routine. To help alleviate some of the time pressure, we bought another car so that Sophie's brother could drive the two of them to school. Taking the car meant that they didn't have to take the school bus and effectively added another 20 minutes to their morning. Even with the car and the home studio, Sophie wakes up at 5:15 a.m. to make sure she does her exercises before school.

What was it like for Sophie to wear a brace? Easy. I was so worried it would be hard, painful, awkward, scary, ugly. It was none of those things. Actually, it was pink. Sophie really did not have an adjustment period wearing her brace. She never had soreness. She never complained about wearing it. She wanted to wear it. She wore it on the beach. She wore it to show rehearsals. She wore it in marching band. She wore it while we vacationed at Disney World. She wore it through airport security (although I don't recommend that one again). She wore it in sleepaway camp. She even wore it on dates. And she did all of this willingly.

Sophie not only wanted to wear her brace, she looked forward to Schroth. It made the scoliosis journey so much easier. Sophie never let her diagnosis get her down. Although my husband and I feel like we've been through the ringer, Sophie never ever did. Certainly she had questions—what kind of pants to wear, what kinds of shirts to wear, whether to tell her friends or not, whether to take it off for gym or not. But she never was negative or upset. Sophie told me she attributed much of her resilience to her previous theater experience. I guess a bunch of auditions without getting the part, or negative feedback from your director builds you up, for the better.

We also learned about Curvy Girls during all of our online research and talk with other parents. The first Curvy Girls' meeting that the three of us attended was cathartic for my husband and me. We were able to acknowledge our guilt, fears, pain, and anxiety. We were able to be teary-eyed in front of others who have done the same.

Nine months after starting to wear her brace, Sophie had her first out-of-brace X-ray. She was instructed to stop wearing her brace for 24 hours and then have an X-ray. At this X-ray, her curves decreased dramatically. What was once 28° and 28° was now 9° and 16°. My husband did a happy dance in the exam room. (Yep, he really did this. I believe "I told you so" was part of the lyrics accompanying the song to his happy dance.") There was no question in our minds that Sophie's curve reduction was due mostly to her dedication to Schroth five days a week and to 22 hours a day of wearing her Rigo brace. From then on, we all were much more relaxed.

For the next X-ray, Sophie stopped wearing her brace for 48 hours prior to the X-ray. Although the curves increased a bit from the prior (but probably within the same range for a manual reading), they were still considerably improved from the initial images. Her curves now measured 15° thoracic and 16° lumbar. These X-rays were taken after approximately one year of wearing her brace, and happened to also correlate with the end of her growth period. Her hand X-rays demonstrated her growth plates had fused. Her height had not changed in six months. Although Sophie was a little disappointed that she was only five feet tall, she also knew this meant that her scoliosis was unlikely to worsen, so she was relieved. Since I am only five feet, one-inch tall, none of us considered five feet to be a shortcoming! The orthopedist told us to start weaning off the brace. We had accomplished so much *with* the brace that it was hard to imagine trying to get rid of it. It was like saying goodbye to an old friend.

I remember reading the first edition of *Straight Talk with the Curvy Girls* book and hearing that scoliosis makes these girls stronger, and that some girls come out on the other side glad that they had scoliosis because it helped define who they are. I remember thinking that I didn't want that. I wanted something else to define my daughter. I did not want her college essay to be about scoliosis. I also remember saying at one of the meetings that I would prefer a really hard exam or SAT test for her to master, and that would be enough of a challenge. I still don't know if I believe that scoliosis made my daughter stronger in the end. But Sophie does believe this. She believes it with all her heart.

I think I have two big take-home messages from this entire experience.

1. We were so lucky to not only have a resilient daughter, but a daughter who embraced her experience. She never had trouble with her brace and really seemed to click with Schroth. She was never ashamed of her brace. For her, no part of this experience was ever negative. There is such a thing as a positive scoliosis experience. There is such a thing as reducing scoliosis curves without surgery, even though it is rarely discussed.
2. Our children are so much more resilient than we expect; they are certainly more resilient than we are as parents.

PART 2

Taking Charge: Teen Talk

A Conversation with Curvy Girls Leah & Rachel

A Message from Leah

I didn't ask for scoliosis; it just happened. You didn't ask to wear a plastic form-fitting back brace, but here it is.

We don't have control over certain things that happen in our lives. As kids and teens with scoliosis, we can feel like we have even less control, which is why it's so important to be able to have a voice in our medical care. There is no such thing as being too young to understand your treatment. While in the doctor's office, even for just a regular check-up, please make your voice heard. If there's something that's not clear, ask. If you have a concern, share. When you are going through something tough, like we are, you need to express yourself.

Make sure the medical staff is not just speaking to your parents **about** you—but that they are talking to you as well! This is YOUR body and you need to know what is going on. Understanding what's happening will make the process much easier and less stressful. When your parents see that you're comfortable, they will feel a little more at ease as well.

I think many of us hold back, scared of what others may think. Remember, taking an active part in your treatment can be very empowering.

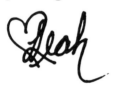

A Message from Rachel

If you are like me, you feel nervous on the drive to your quarterly check-up. The anxiety of seeing my doctor, and not knowing what the outcome would be, always left me worried.

Throughout my scoliosis journey, I allowed the results of my X-rays to dictate my self-esteem and determine how I measured "success." If my curves worsened, I thought I "failed" bracing or my Schroth Method exercises. During these years I put an enormous amount of pressure on myself, which was both unrealistic and unfair.

If I could go back in time and give one piece of advice to my 11-year-old self, it would be this: The numeric value of your curve degree does NOT define you.

The last thing I want is another young girl or boy to feel that same kind of burden. So, I am asking you to please be kinder and have more patience with yourself during your scoliosis journey. Be proud of yourself for wearing your brace. Be proud that you did everything you could if surgery becomes your outcome. We need to stop shaming ourselves when things do not go as planned, and realize that it is okay to be perfectly imperfect.

Remember, an X-ray will only generate a number; however, it is up to you to determine how that number will impact you. Do not allow a number to make you feel less than.

Rachel

Embracing Fashion

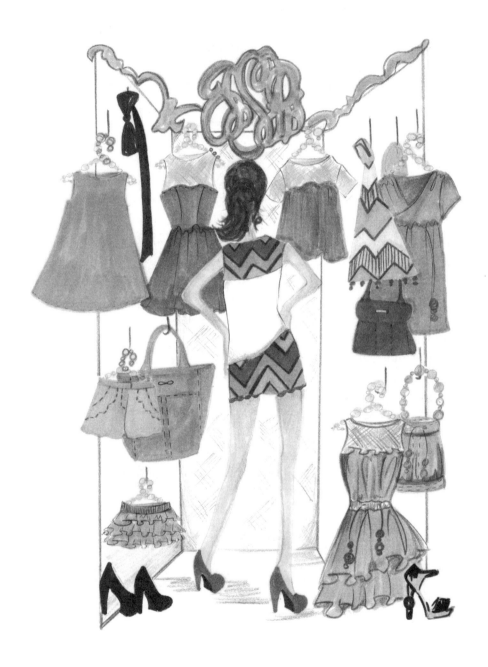

RACHEL'S SHOPPING TIPS

As a teenage girl who wore a back brace throughout middle school, I understand how overwhelming it can be finding clothes that complement your back brace. This part of the book is designed to help each individual girl feel confident and beautiful in her brace.

BECOMING A FASHIONISTA

I want to start off by reassuring you that finding clothes to wear with your brace is so much easier than you might think. When I wore my brace the biggest fashion trends were skinny jeans and tightly fitted crop-tops, which are not ideal for bracing. Thankfully, today's clothing stores carry a variety of options to complement your brace!

By the end of this section, I hope all of you will not only feel like fashionistas, but also have fun while shopping for your back brace!

FALL & WINTER

I personally love to shop for these seasons because there are more options to choose from. You can wear anything from stylishly oversized and long sweaters, leather/denim jackets, cardigans, to knitted sweatshirts. There are also hoodies, pullover sweatshirts and vests. Another great option is plaid shirts. These tops come in many color patterns and can be worn two ways: by itself or by layering them with a t-shirt or tank-top underneath. All of these items mentioned are a part of every girls' wardrobe, not just the ones who are looking for tops to wear with their back brace.

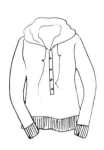 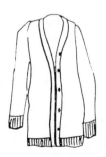 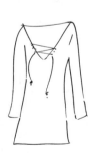 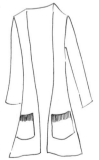

SPRING & SUMMER
Trendy Tops for Bracing

A lot of girls have asked questions about how to dress with their back brace in warmer weather. Their number one concern is becoming overheated. Fortunately, there are amazing styles to choose from with some helpful tricks to stay cool!

The primary goal is looking for tops that are loose fitting or have a slight flare. Shirts such as baby doll tops and oversized graphic t-shirts are perfect wardrobe accessories for girls wearing a brace. They will not cling or stick to you—and if you choose to wear a more fitting shirt, layering will be key.

Materials such as nylon/spandex are also great alternatives. Try to find camisoles that have no seams; they are more comfortable and do not leave any imprints on your skin.

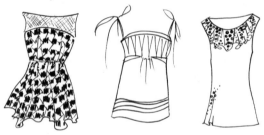

Shopping for Dresses and Skirts...

Sundresses, T-shirt dresses, and flowy maxi dresses are just a few examples of the great options you have! While shopping for dresses, I recommend avoiding any material that is thin. Sometimes those thinly made dresses (and shirts, too) will rip and develop little holes from our straps.

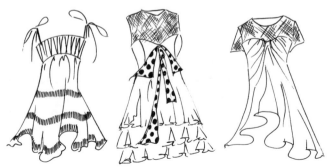

Skirts are extremely useful because they are easy to wear over your brace. The best kinds are the flare-out, ruffled ones. You should avoid pencil skirts because they are too tight and have a tendency of showing the bulkiness of your brace.

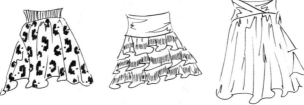

Fun Tricks

One of our Curvy Girls' members shared this tip for those hot summer days. She took her brace off and let it sit in her freezer for 15 minutes. When she put it back on, it felt cool and refreshing against her body. If your brace cannot fit in the freezer, many girls put their undershirt in a Ziplock bag in the freezer for a few minutes!

ALL YEAR LONG
Jeans, Jeggings, and More…

When choosing jeans, girls always ask, "What is more comfortable—wearing jeans tucked inside the brace, or going up a size to put the bottoms over the brace?" This is a personal choice, but I chose to wear mine over my brace. If this is something you do not feel comfortable doing, there is another solution—jeggings! Jeggings are excellent jean replacements. They are essentially leggings, but have an exterior print that replicates jeans! You no longer need to buy jeans that are a size too big or feel uncomfortable tucking your normal size denim pants under the brace. They are made with elastic material and they stretch to fit all types of figures. They are comfortable, affordable, and fashionable. Sweatpants, gym shorts, leggings, and yoga pants also offer girls alternative options for comfort in the brace.

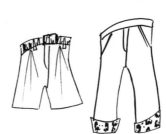
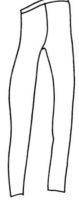

SCARVES

Scarves are perfect for girls whose back brace has a shoulder strap!

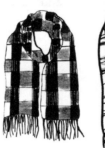
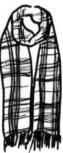

Have fun when choosing these items; and more importantly, do not be afraid to experiment and see what works best for you!

FINAL THOUGHTS

Never forget, if you are having a hard time finding clothes to complement the brace, there is nothing wrong with wearing your brace on the outside of your clothes! It is one of the most empowering things you can do for yourself and your curvy girl friends. By doing this, you are raising scoliosis awareness in the most amazing way!

A Brace... Are They Crazy?

Why do we have to wear a back brace?

From two girls who have been braced for years, let us tell you why bracing is important. The brace is designed to help maintain and control the progression of your curves. If we do not wear our brace, the curves will more than likely progress. Our biggest growth spurt occurs during our adolescent years. For someone with scoliosis, this is also the time when our curves can progress the most.

How do we know that bracing really works?

This is a great question. In 2014, a four-year study known as BrAIST, concluded bracing was not only effective, but the more hours you wore your brace the higher the success rate. So yes, we really do know that bracing works.

What does it feel like to wear a back brace?

We like to compare adjusting to a back brace to getting used to orthodontic braces. Remember that restricted, tight feeling on your teeth when they were first put on? Remember how sore your mouth was until your teeth adjusted to the hardware? And yet a week later, you were back to eating whatever you wanted. That same reaction will occur with your back brace. The more you wear it, the easier it will get.

Does it hurt to wear a back brace?

It is uncomfortable at first to wear the back brace because the brace is actually supporting your body in a more balanced position. For some, it might actually feel a little painful because your body is used to being pulled towards the dominant curve side, and the brace is trying to change that. Your body feels weird since it is actually being put into alignment for the first time, which is why the brace initially feels uncomfortable. Again, it will get better the more you wear the brace.

How tight does the brace have to be?

Did you ever see a person wear loose braces on their teeth? Well the same rule applies to our back braces. In order for our back brace to be doing its job, it should be worn snug and tight. Your hands should not be able to slip down into your brace. However, you do not want to wear it too tight initially as that will make your adjustment to bracing more difficult. Your best bet is to ask your orthotist to put a mark on your straps to indicate the ideal position to where the straps should be tightened.

How will I know the difference between what is considered normal discomfort and pain that I should tell my parent or doctor about?

Some tenderness is normal. Remember, the brace is trying to resist the natural curve of your body. But if your skin begins to bruise, redness does not go away, or you feel sharp pains going down your leg or around your abdomen, then it is time to tell your parent and orthotist. None of these symptoms are acceptable because bracing should not be causing significant pain or bruising. Your parents need to contact your orthotist to find out what is causing the problem.

Do I have to wear the brace every day? Is it bad if sometimes I cheat a little?

Yes, you have to wear the brace every day. Brace compliance is very important. And yes, you can cheat, but try to make up for the hours out of brace. The bottom line is that you are only hurting yourself by not complying with the hours that your doctor has set. Always ask yourself, "Is this worth it?" You do not want to regret your decision years down the road. And remember, if we took off our orthodontic braces whenever we wanted to, our teeth would never have good results.

What do you recommend wearing under my brace?

Most girls like the non-ribbed, cotton boy's sleeveless undershirts. Wearing this shirt under your brace adds comfort and prevents the skin from having direct contact with the brace.

Two online brace shirt companies we are familiar with are braceforstyle.com and hopescloset.com.

I sometimes feel sharp edges around my brace. What causes this?

If the sharp edges are from the padding wearing down, congratulations, this means that you are consistently wearing your brace! Once again, let your parents know what is going on. They will need to make an appointment with the orthotist.

More than likely the orthotist will need to add some padding around the edges of your brace. In the meantime, purchase some moleskin at a local pharmacy. Have your parents cut and place the moleskin in the areas that are sharp until you are able to have your orthotist make the necessary adjustments.

What can be done about the holes in my shirts from the metal on the brace?

Haven't we told you about shopping for new clothes?! You will need to go shopping to buy clothes that work best with your brace. When you shop for clothes, make sure to choose sturdy material. Also, put moleskin over the metal parts of the brace. Be prepared to replace the moleskin periodically because it will fall off.

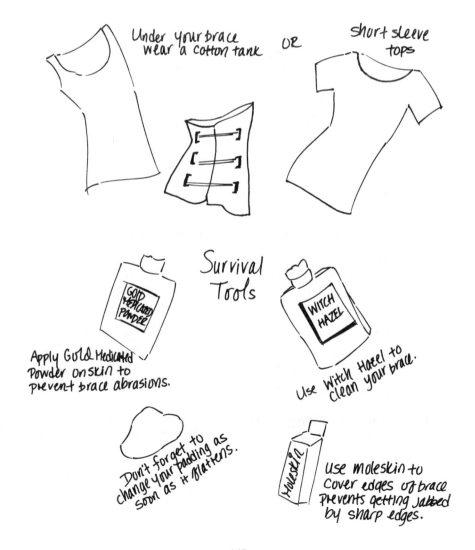

How can I keep my brace clean?

We wiped our braces down with household cleansers like Fantastik® and Formula 409®.

How can you sleep with a back brace?

Leah shared this tip during one of our first support group meetings. Her trick was to put a pillow or two in between her legs to balance out the unevenness in her hips. This little trick may help you get a better night's sleep. Another great tip is to purchase a foam mattress pad topper; the more padding the better for extra support and comfort.

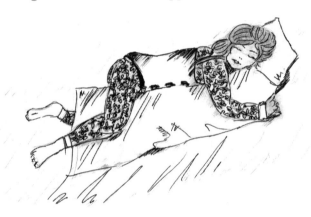

I'm nervous my friends will find out I am wearing a back brace. Any advice on what to do?

Yes. Tell your friends. We know you are scared; we have all been there. Keeping it a secret makes it worse. It will be so much easier on you to tell them the truth. You will be surprised how supportive they can be. They will probably have a ton of questions for you, but this is because they do not understand what you are going through. Honestly and patiently explain to them what scoliosis is and what the brace is doing. This will help them understand and better support you.

Can I wear my brace during activities?

That depends on the activity. Your back brace is *not* worn for running, participating in gym class, dance classes, or other sports, and certainly not swimming. Doing these activities while wearing your brace could actually hurt you. If you are not sure whether or not you should wear your back brace, it is always best to ask your doctor.

Do I have to shower with my brace on?
No. You do not shower, bathe or swim with your brace on. Showering and swimming are brace-free time!

Is it normal to have bruises from my brace?
Absolutely NOT. If you are bruising, tell your parents.

How long does it take to get used to wearing the brace?
A well-made brace should take about a week to get used to.

How many hours do I have to wear this brace?
That will depend on your orthopedic doctor. Leah wore her brace for twenty-two hours a day, while Rachel's orthopedic doctor instructed her to wear it for sixteen hours.

Will I ever like wearing my brace?
That is up to you. As much as you may dislike your back brace in the beginning, it will be easier on you if you change your feelings about your brace. Always remember that your back brace is there for a reason. It is protecting you by fighting against the curves in your spine. Maintaining a positive mental attitude, "I will get through this," will help make life easier.

Do you have any suggestions to help motivate me to wear my brace?
We know that wearing your brace from 16 to as many as 22 hours a day can be a real challenge. There are a variety of ways to potentially help you stay motivated. For example, consider using a "reward chart" in which you record your brace-wearing hours every day and then reward yourself with something you like at the end of a set period of time (a day, week, or month). Some girls create a reward chart with their parents. Or, you can consider tracking your time in an app on your smartphone. One we are familiar with is called BraceTrack.

School Nurse Letter

After listening to Curvy Girls talk about the difficulty they have with bracing in school, we put together a letter that Curvy Girls can give to school nurses to help them understand what we are going through and how important their role is in our lives. You may want to use this letter at your school.

Visit straighttalkscoliosis.com to download a copy.

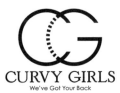

CURVY GIRLS
We've Got Your Back

International Scoliosis Support Groups
Leah Stoltz, Founder 2006
www.curvygirlsscoliosis.com

Dear School Nurse,

This letter is to share with you my experience having scoliosis, and offer some ideas on how you can help other affected students deal with their everyday challenges. When I was diagnosed and endured three years of bracing and, ultimately, major spine surgery, it was my School Nurse and Physical Education teacher who made a tremendous difference in my school adjustment. My School Nurse's office was a safe place to remove my brace and store it during gym glass. She reassured me that I could ask her for assistance at any time; I felt that she was very sensitive toward my condition.

It's very important to realize that, aside from being a medical condition, scoliosis affects us most emotionally. Kids in middle school try very hard to feel like they fit in. Wearing this uncomfortable contraption to school every day poses some very embarrassing situations that can become more traumatic than most people realize. Oftentimes, kids with scoliosis try very hard to keep their disease a secret from peers, which can result in emotional stress.

Kids with scoliosis frequently face challenges such as:

- *Acute self-consciousness around body image and braces*
- *Avoidance of situations (gym class, swimming pools, school dances, and proms) where the secret of the brace or their scoliosis might be exposed*
- *Fear of facing major spine surgery*

Students with scoliosis need to feel that they have an ally in the school. You can help the student with their adjustment in many ways such as:

1. *Ensure that they have a person to seek out, and a private space where they can remove, hide, or store their brace, so that they can avoid questions from their peers;*

2. *Communicate the student's needs and concerns to other school personnel, such as late passes and additional set of textbooks (to reduce carrying a heavy load);*

3. *Make sure that scoliosis is discussed in health classes;*

4. *Connect the student with counseling services if they show signs of anxiety or depression.*

It's very important that the school be sensitive to children who are being braced for scoliosis and possibly facing surgery. Your acceptance and attitude towards your student can make a world of difference. I know, because they made a difference for me!

Thank you for your consideration.

Sincerely,

Leah Stoltz, Founder

Bone Nutrition Trivia

If you have scoliosis, you can't afford to compromise the health of your bones any further. You need to be especially mindful of avoiding products that deplete your supply of calcium.

Robyn Rexford is an nutritionist who shares some interesting facts with the Curvy Girls:

DID YOU KNOW?

- Caffeine, an ingredient in soda, depletes calcium, which then weakens our bones.
- Caffeine depletes bone density. To reduce the risk of osteoporosis later in life, it is crucial that females in their teens and twenties build up bone mass.
- If you are anticipating spinal fusion surgery, it is most important to make sure that your bones are in the best shape possible.
- A 2016 study concluded that daily calcium and vitamin D3 improves low bone mass and may positively improve adolescent idiopathic scoliosis curve progression in patients.
- Orthopedic surgeons are now prescribing calcium and vitamin D3 supplements as part of their treatment plans for AIS patients.
- Milk contains calcium to build bones. The only significant difference between skim and whole milk is FAT content. The difference in calcium content is negligible. So, the only thing you get more of by drinking whole milk is fat.
- The best drink you can have is water-water-water—or low-fat milk!
- One of the main ingredients in cola is phosphoric acid.
- Dark soda (cola) can clean your porcelain toilet, remove corrosion off car battery terminals, and clean blood from accident scenes. And yet, this is what we drink!

Leah's Surgery Tips

You know what is best for you. Speak up to make people aware of how you feel or what you need. Here are some suggestions:

- I found it helpful to be **distracted the night before** and asked my parents to have a sleepover with my best friend.

- You'll want your **hair away from your face**, or pulled back, because you won't be able to wash it for a few days. I know a couple of girls who had their hair cut shorter in order to make it easier to deal with during recovery. Curvy Girl Rachel and her older sister came over the night before surgery to French braid my hair. The braid kept my hair in place.

- **No-rinse shampoo cap** since you won't be able to wash your hair

- If you wear **glasses,** make sure you like them as there's no way you're going to want to put your contacts in.

- It's not necessary to buy new **sleepwear.** Believe it or not, the open-back hospital gowns are the best to wear as they are comfortable and allow easy access for the doctors and nurses. You won't want to pull anything over your head because it's difficult to raise your arms up. Just make sure someone holds your gown closed when you are walking the halls or put on sweatpants. Better yet, put another hospital gown on like a robe!

- You may want to **pack your own** pillow, fuzzy blanket, large sweats or oversized tee shirt, slippers, headphones, cell phone/iPad and charger, and anything that helps you relax.

- Use **cups with built-in straw**

- Some girls want to have friends and family **visit** them in the hospital, and some are against it. Make sure that you verbalize your desire to your parents and other people. This is **YOUR recovery time** and you need to be as comfortable as possible. You don't want to be feeling miserable in the hospital, and on top of that, feel like you have to socialize with visitors. Personally, I loved having people visit, even though I felt embarrassed about how I looked. They helped me take my mind off of things and broke the monotony of only seeing the nurses, my parents, and my brother.

- Having a **positive attitude** is important going into surgery. Positive thoughts help to accelerate healing. There are plenty of meditation apps that can help with staying calm or relaxing, both before and after surgery.

- Period Panties. Even if you are not expecting to get **your period** during your time in the hospital, it could still happen. I couldn't believe it when I got my period the night before my surgery. My pediatric intensive care nurse said, "I know it seems like a cruel joke but probably 75% of girls will get their period." This is possibly your body's response to the stress of going for surgery. You may want to pack your preferred products.

- I was surprised that I had NO **attention span** to read anything. I mostly just flipped through magazines to see the pictures and watched TV. I couldn't concentrate, which was probably a factor of anesthesia and post-surgery medications.

- Don't be frightened when you see your **face after surgery.** My eyes and face were pretty puffy from being face down for so long.

- One of our biggest fears is about **pain after surgery.** My nurse said it best, "Pain is to be managed." This is done with oral medication and a medicine pump. You will repeatedly be asked for your "pain number." This is a 1-10 scale: 0 being pain-free and 10 being the worst. You need to speak up if you are in any pain.

    You will be given a **medicine pump** after surgery; don't be afraid to use it! The pump is programmed to only give safe doses of medication based on your weight. You CANNOT overdose and will not become addicted in such a short period of time. So, press the button when you feel the slightest pain.

- Press a small pillow over your stomach when you **cough or sneeze**.

- **Avoid** sitting on a **soft chair or couch**; it can be difficult to get up.

- You **go home** when your pain is under control, you can walk around, manage stairs, and eat regular food.

- Anesthesia, pain medications, reduced food and fluid intake slow your system down, which can cause **constipation**. It helps to drink plenty of water. If you are constipated, ask the nurse for a stool softener.

- It's important to **protect your healing scar** from the sun by keeping the area covered. Remember to wait until your surgeon gives you the go ahead before using sunscreen on your scar.

- My **scar/incision** area felt **itchy** for a while after surgery. This is part of the healing process, but unfortunately, it's uncomfortable to itch because of the area feeling numb. It helps to apply lotion, aloe, or a cool compress to distract and relieve the feeling.

- It's important to have a **good relationship with your surgeon**. I was lucky to have a great relationship with my doctor and, therefore, trusted him to know everything would be OK. I'm happy to say I still keep in touch with him to this day.

- And when you're ready, **show off your scar!!** Be proud of overcoming the surgery and everything you've done to get to where you are.

MOM'S TIPS

- **Watch the Nutrition:** Getting your body into the best possible condition will help in your recovery process. Eating balanced meals creates a healthy body that promotes healing. Antioxidant rich foods such as berries can aid in the healing process. Papaya and kiwi are rich in zinc, which helps build your immune system. Don't forget to drink plenty of water leading up to and after surgery in order to cleanse your body.

    You will want to limit the intake of synthetic sugar (especially high fructose corn syrup), because the excess intake of sugar affects our immune system.

- **Mind the Medication:** Ibuprofen (Motrin®, Advil®, certain menstrual pain medications) is not to be taken three- to six-months prior to fusion surgery and up until your physician says your spine is fully fused. Because ibuprofen interferes with blood clotting, it can interfere with the fusion process. So it's important to check with your surgeon's office before taking prescribed or over-the-counter medication, or any type of herbal supplements.

- **Strengthen your Core:** Core exercises are good for everyone but will especially help you with your post-surgery movement. The stronger your stomach muscles, the less stress on your back muscles.

  Have you ever rolled sideways down a hill for fun? This is called a "logroll" and is just what you need to be able to do after surgery to help you get out of bed. (Well, not the rolling down the hill part!) While at home, practice turning from your back to your side as if you were a log. This means keeping your body stiff like a wood log, while turning your whole body as one unit from your back to your side. No body part turns without the other parts. By maintaining equal distribution from your feet to your head, you will not be using back muscles to turn. Whenever you change positions, tighten your abdominal muscles.

  An easy way to tighten ab muscles is by taking a breath in and then slowly letting it out while pulling your belly button in toward your spine. Practice this when getting out of bed each morning, and it will be easier to do after surgery.

  After you have rolled onto your side, slowly scoot to the edge of the bed and put your legs over the edge. Use your arms to support yourself while sitting up.

  So let's strengthen your arm muscles, and while you're at it, how about those thigh muscles to help you on and off chairs and ... the toilet too!

- **Practice Positive Mindset:** Have you heard the saying "mind-over-matter?" Taking control over how you think about something can impact the outcome. Practicing a positive mindset is proven to be a key factor in reducing stress. In turn, reducing stress will have a positive impact post-surgery, leading to a faster recovery.

  One way to practice a positive mindset is by visualizing positive outcomes. Keep a journal and write down the positive results you anticipate from your surgery. For example, "I will be two inches taller. I will no longer have pain."

When scary or negative thoughts come to your mind, remind yourself or reread what you wrote. Allow the positive surgery outcomes to become your focus.

You will want to acknowledge those negative or scary thoughts by saying, "There's that thought" and then visualize it floating away in a cloud. Repeat this technique each time you have an unwelcome thought.

Surrounding yourself with positive images pre- and post-surgery is key to creating a positive mindset. A fun activity used to reinforce this is a vision board—a collection of images you find that reflect the goals that you would like to achieve. Place your vision board where you can see it most often. Many girls have it in their bedrooms. By having it in a set location in their room, it's the first thing they see in the morning and the last thing they see before going to bed. What better way to remind yourself what you're trying to achieve!

And lastly, it's important to surround yourself with people who are encouraging and supportive about your surgery.

Taking "Back" Control

Rachel Mulvaney

After nearly two years being out of my brace, my curves increased from 33° to 42° and I was living in chronic back pain. While doing research for our first book, we came across a European-based treatment called the Schroth Method which appeared to be very promising. This method teaches specific exercises that might stop or reverse curves from progressing. With spinal fusion now being considered, this treatment became my last opportunity to avoid surgery.

In 2010, my mother and I went to Stevens Point, Wisconsin for a two-week intensive program to learn these exercises. During this time, I wrote a daily blog and posted it on the Curvy Girls' online forum. While I was 15 years old at the time, this experience left a lifechanging impact on me. What follows is my journey at Scoliosis rehab and the lessons I learned.

AN INSIDER'S LOOK AT THE SCHROTH METHOD

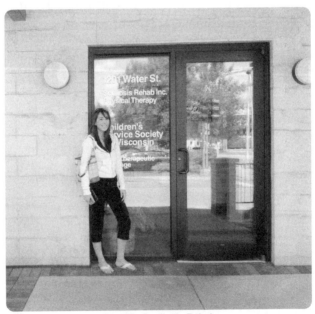

Outside Scoliosis Rehab

DAY 1

Don't let the smile fool you; I was quite nervous before I walked through these doors. Once I did, I was greeted by the most dedicated and passionate group of people I've ever met.

My first day started off with a review about myself—what activities I like to do, and generally getting a little history on my scoliosis. Because every curve is different, it is important for the physical therapists to know what type of activities we do. By learning this information, they are able to correct and suggest an alternative way to do our activities without our bodies collapsing into our curves.

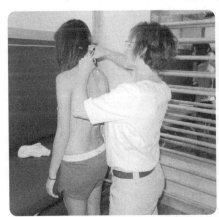
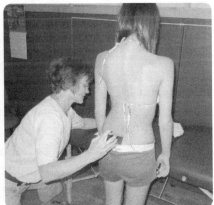

First day at Scoliosis Rehab

Beth Janssen (above) takes my measurements and later tests my strength and flexibility.

Later on, Beth reviews my X-rays and we learn that I have three curves, not two, which means I will need five pelvic corrections to keep my body in alignment. I ended the first day by learning a new breathing technique.

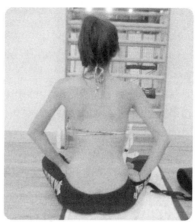
Elongating pose and Schroth pose

DAY 2

Hey everyone, day two in rehab and I thought I should share some information I learned today. If you get muscle spasms, this will explain it all!

Since scoliosis forces our curves to grow towards one side more than the other, it causes the muscles in our backs to be in an imbalanced position. The curvature development and rotational pull of the spine will lead to collapsed areas and unevenness in our bodies. The muscles on the concave (curving inward) side are shortened, and on the convex (curving outward, bulging) part of the back, the muscles are stretched out and elongated. Due to the muscles having different resting lengths, they cannot have equal activation; therefore, it can create back pain and muscle spasms. So what we worked on today was learning how to shift my body into a position that decreased the pressure on my muscles that are close to my large curve.

DAYS 3 & 4

Today was the first day that I was able to walk in alignment. It felt weird—but it was a great feeling to see that when I looked in the mirror, I was straight for the first time!

Part 2: Taking Charge

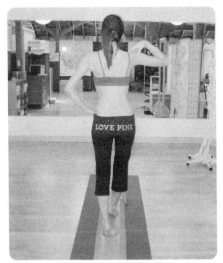

Getting myself aligned with the Schroth Walk

By the third day the amount of change I see in my body is crazy. I feel myself getting stronger and can feel the difference from within.

One of the exercises I am currently doing is training my breathing. We're working on expanding the concave side of my rib cage where the collapse of my curve is. By breathing into my weak spot and my weak side, it literally puts my spine in a straight position.

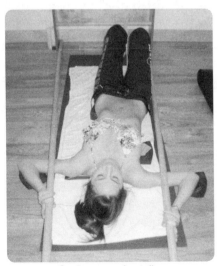

Supine - growing taller

Here I am working on how to grow taller, which is called "elongate."

One technique of elongating is by using straps to put on my waist, which we then attach to a bar. I lay on the floor with a small beanbag under my left hip, one under my right rib cage/shoulder blade, and another under my left shoulder. We use these to untwist the rotation. I continue to breathe deeply. As I do so, I'm using the muscles in my ribs to grow taller and taller with each breath. Along with this, I'm expanding my right rib cage, which will symmetrically balance my rib cages. I literally feel my spine being pulled straight just by the power of my breath.

DAY 5

On Friday I begin to do the exercises more independently. Instead of having my physical therapists help me elongate, I can do it on my own. I'm becoming more aware of where my body is in space. In other words, when I'm not doing my exercises and my body is no longer in the correct position, I've noticed that I collapse into my curve way too much. We have habits like slouching and not sitting in good posture throughout our lives, and it's hard to break these bad habits. However, little do we know that when we have scoliosis and we slouch, we're doing much more than just collapsing into our curves; we're also causing damage to the discs in our backs. How are they becoming damaged? Well, when we slouch, it puts pressure on the discs. When these discs are completely squished it's called a "herniated disc" and pain will be constant. One of the best things about this clinic is how much education you receive. I am taught all about the development of my curves, what causes my pain, and now, what I can do to prevent it.

Part 2: Taking Charge

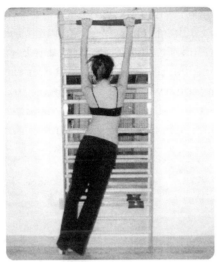
Pendulum

The above exercise is called "Pendulum," where I go on the top bar of the wallboard and swing. The more I work on doing these exercises, the better I get at it. On the first day I was capable of only doing four or five. Now I'm up to thirty on day five. I can breathe longer and elongate better too! On Monday, I'll be working on doing more exercises on my own, so I'll let you all know how that goes. I am so surprised about how much I'm able to do. I'm doing things that I never thought I was capable of doing because I was always in pain.

DAYS 6 & 7

I'll be combining both days six and seven because I haven't necessarily done anything new. The difference between the end of my first week and the beginning of my second is that I am able to do everything more independently. I now know how to put my body in alignment, as well as perform the exercises on my own with very few corrections from the therapist. I am slowly beginning to see all the changes that my body is doing. One of the things that stood out the most in this journey occurred on day six.

I was doing an exercise called "Side Laying." The position for that is laying on my left side with a cushion under my left hip, left shoulder, and a pad for my head. As I breathe deeply, I try to open up the weak side (left rib cage), weak spot (under my right rib cage), and push my right rib cage forward. While I was doing that, I heard my mom and Beth in awe of my results. Feeling frustrated that I could not internally feel what they were physically seeing, Beth ran her fingers down each vertebrae of my spine. For my whole life, all I ever experienced when my doctor examined my spine was his hands swirling in different directions. However, today for the first time, someone's hands went down my back in a straight line. Beth then moved a mirror into position so I was able to see it with my own eyes, as well as feel it. It was a great day!

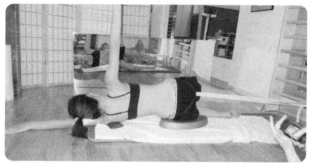

Side Laying

DAYS 8 & 9

I cannot believe my time here is coming to an end, and to be honest, I am shocked that it has gone so fast. Much of my time now is spent perfecting the exercises that I've already been taught.

On Wednesday, I was taught something new—the proper way to work out my abdominals. First, Beth asked me to show her how I normally would exercise my abs. Excitedly, I laid on the ground and proceeded to demonstrate my favorite double leg lifts. For those of you who aren't sure what this exercise is, allow me to explain. You lie on the ground and swiftly raise your legs up in a 45° angle. You then slowly bring your legs down as low as you can and then split them apart, bring them back together, hold them for a few seconds (or as long as you can), bring your legs back up to that 45° angle, and then repeat the pattern about 25 times.

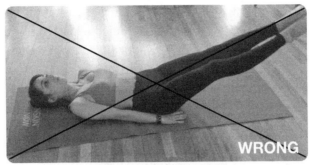

Improper abdominal excercise

After I demonstrated this exercise, Beth looked at me and asked, "Who taught you this exercise?" I told her that it was part of my warm-up exercises when I was taking dance for nine years. She then asked me never to do them again and explained how much damage I was doing to the already pressured discs in my spine. I would later learn that by doing double leg lifts, you're not giving your back the support it needs. The main problem when doing these leg lifts is that your back arches too much (increasing your lordosis), which would make it very difficult to maintain your pelvic corrections.

Beth then promised that the exercises she would be giving me would not only be safe for my spine, but would create the six-pack abs of my dreams.

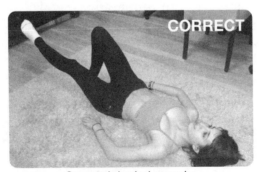

Correct abdominal excercise

By keeping one foot bent on the floor and the other raised, I am able to keep my back in a more stabilized position. Just as we would do in our normal pelvic correction, you give yourself slight lordosis and from that position you are able to control the way your hips shift. Also, when using one leg at a time, you're not increasing the rotation in your spine, something that is essential to avoid for someone with scoliosis.

After one afternoon of doing these "new and improved" ab exercises, my stomach felt like a rock. And the best part is they are actually easier than the ones I learned years ago in my dance classes.

On day nine, I was doing the exercises independently while Beth observed and corrected me when it was needed. Before I left this afternoon, Beth gave me a book with a typed-up description of every exercise I've learned in the past two weeks, along with a picture of me doing the exercise as a reminder of what my body has to look like while doing them. I have nearly perfected each task and I am eager to say that I will be returning here next year to challenge myself and get new exercises to work on.

I truly hope one day soon that the scoliosis-specific exercises will change the way doctors view scoliosis in this country. In my opinion, these exercises should be one of the first things offered to a child and their parents. I understand this is a lifestyle change, but trust me when I say it's worth it.

As a teenager, when we hear the word "forever," we either don't know what to expect, or freak out due to the thought of how big the time span is. I was told that within a month or two these exercises would be easier for me. Well, I'm on week two and I've already adapted to these changes.

I came here suffering with pain nearly every day for five years, and now the only time I truly have pain is when my body is out of neutral, meaning my pelvis is out of balance and rotated.

LAST DAY AT SCOLIOSIS REHAB

When I first arrived at Scoliosis Rehab, I was both skeptical and nervous. Being the first one in our support group to try this type of treatment, I was excited but still scared. I worried about whether these exercises would really help me, would I be able to do the exercises, and mostly, would I continue to do them? After it was all done, I told my mom that I owe the girls in our support group my honest feelings about the experience here. Learning these exercises was a lot of hard work, but it was *not* harder than learning to adapt to wearing a back brace for sixteen hours a day for nearly three years.

Are the exercises the same for all scoliosis patients? No. Similar to how no curves are the same, neither are exercises prescribed to each person. The treatment is about providing you with tools to help your scoliosis. Can this method guarantee scoliosis will not progress? No. There will always be curves that progress no matter what preventions we take; however, learning these exercises will never be a waste of time for you.

I've been in everyone's shoes with regard to bracing and doctor visits every four- to six-months. Each visit, when I'd go in for my X-rays (just like you guys do today), the doctor would examine my back and I'd literally hold my breath until he would announce whether my curve progressed or not. It was the worst feeling in the world, feeling this helpless, even though I did everything I was asked to do. But after nearly five years, I don't have to feel this pressure or the frustration of feeling powerless. For the first time since I was eleven and put into a back brace, I feel like I have taken back what I had lost—control over my own body. For five years, I complained to many doctors about back, shoulder, and hip pain, and no one truly believed me. But these therapists understood my pain.

After just three days of being here, my pain was getting less and less. Today, I'm leaving totally pain-free thanks to the invaluable lessons I've learned. My only real regret is wishing I had known about this method of exercise while my spine was still growing.

The team at the facility also took great pains to ensure that I'd be able to remember precisely how to do my exercises once I got home. I would leave Scoliosis Rehab with a videotape of myself performing each exercise. Beth did a voice-over on the tape, reinforcing what I need to be striving for in order to execute each position to the highest benefit for my body.

My goal is to be able to do each position well and be able to maintain this position for about five minutes. This isn't such a terrible goal to strive for, especially if you're doing these exercises while listening to music. I have absolutely no regrets of giving up two weeks of my summer vacation to go to Scoliosis Rehab. The tools I have learned, I hope to carry with me for the rest of my life.

Was it hard work? Yes, but now ask me, "Was it worth it?" Absolutely! Look at my results. Now you decide.

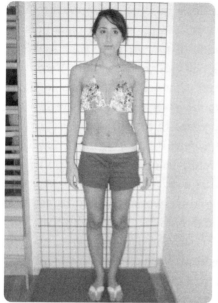 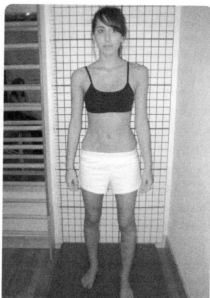

First day at the Scoliosis Rehab   Two weeks later

As you can see my shoulders are level, my hips are more centered, and my overall posture is entirely different than it was at the start. Notice my right foot is slightly behind my left foot. That change allowed me to even out my hips, which gave me my new postural position.

AFTER SCOLIOSIS REHAB—16 YEARS OLD

Four months later, I had my first follow-up visit with my orthopedic doctor since my return from the Scoliosis Rehab clinic. For the first time in five years, I was not in pain. After a brief conversation regarding my experiences at the clinic, Dr. Labiak began my examination. I stood up, bent forward, and he placed the scoliometer on my back. As he wrote down the information in my chart, my mom asked if he noticed a change. He smiled and said, "Yes. If Rachel were to have a scoliosis school screening tomorrow, she would pass."

"What does that mean?" my mother asked.

"When the kids go in for their school screening exams, a scoliometer reading of 5 to 7 is considered within normal range; Rachel is now a 7!" the doctor explained. He reminded me that this does not necessarily mean that the measurement of my curve (Cobb angle) is different.

"That is something we won't know until your X-rays in five months."

By then, it would have been a year since my last X-rays were taken and I would have been doing this method of exercises for eight full months. As an added bonus, we found an old orthopedic evaluation form dated two years prior showing a scoliometer exam score of my ATR (angle of trunk rotation), and it was a 15. That's quite a difference!

Five months later, we returned to take new X-rays. As we waited anxiously to find out if the exercises had helped to hold my curve from progressing, Dr. Labiak began to mark and measure my curves on the images. It seemed like forever, and then he finally announced that my thoracic curve was 30°! I was shocked and wanted to scream, but knew this wasn't the place. My curve decreased 12°! My lumbar curve went from 26° to 22° I think Dr. Labiak was as shocked as we were. He continued to compare both X-rays and concluded that technically this shouldn't have happened to a child who has been skeletally mature for two and a half years. Dr. Labiak was very happy for me. I just hope that he will tell his other patients about this treatment.

The reduction in my curves fuels me to continue exercising five days a week, twenty- to thirty-minutes a day. My new posture has become second nature. The point of doing the exercises is to make the muscles strong enough to maintain "correction" all the time. It's like having an internal brace. Sometimes I chuckle to myself when I am asked when I had surgery. But it frustrates me when I hear that my corrections are not accurate because I stood in my pelvic corrections for my X-rays. Why wouldn't I when I hold my body this way all the time? So, when my X-rays are taken, or when I'm sitting, walking or standing, I remain in that same position—neutral.

TWO YEARS LATER: 18 YEARS OLD

I felt like I was 13 years old again, as I nervously waited in my orthopedic surgeons office for the first set of X-rays in two years. My doctor came in holding my X-rays in his hands and he immediately walked over to put the film on the screen to review together.

He spoke, but I did not hear a word he said, because my eyes immediately went straight towards the numeric measurements marked on my spine. It read, 22 thoracic, 17 lumbar.

I could not help but cry because it showed me that after all that hard work, it finally paid off. I accomplished something that statistically should not have happened—decreased my curve by 50% without needing surgery.

Sometimes it's hard to process, but three years prior we were discussing surgery because my curves were progressing and my back pain was intolerable. However, I am here to attest that learning these excercises has changed the quality of my life for the absolute best.

This treatment has given me a gift that no one else could have ever provided me with: control over my scoliosis. It has made me realize that all of us have the power to start over, and redirect the curves life throws at us.

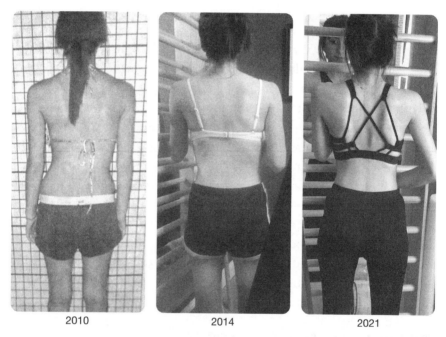

| 2010 | 2014 | 2021 |

I am proud to say it has been over eleven years and I still practice my scoliosis-specific exercises. The Schroth-based exercises continue to greatly impact my life and I am excited to share my experiences with other families. I have dedicated the past decade to raising awareness on the powerful effects scoliosis-specific exercises can offer. It is my hope that my story will motivate someone to never give up, despite the odds they are up against.

Curvy Girls has always been an incredible support system throughout my scoliosis journey. Whether I needed help finding clothes to wear for my brace or the confidence to tell my classmates about my condition, there was always someone to turn to. However, when I learned these new exercises, I could not ask my peers for support, as I was the first girl in our group (and organization) to start this treatment. For this reason, I wrote my experiences on the Curvy Girls' forum page for all to see. My intention was to create a resource that would help others feel more prepared before learning this program.

After posting my journey online, many families across the country reached out for more information. Below are the most commonly asked questions I've received from girls and parents:

What was the hardest part for you while learning these exercises?

Believe it or not, learning those deep breathings from my diaphragm was the hardest part! Initially, it was very difficult to visualize how to take those big breaths while activating muscles that needed to be moved.

What helped you improve your deep breathing techniques while exercising?

Through the power of her words, Beth often used imagery and metaphors to help connect how and where I needed to activate specific muscles. She told to me think of my torso as a balloon being pumped with air, and to pretend the muscles in my stomach were like a zipper.

It may sound silly, but when you are expanding the "balloon" through those deep breathings, it helped me envision the power of my breath. Beth would instruct me to exhale slowly, and to pull my core muscles in my stomach in an upward motion like a zipper on my pants. Without an exaggeration, I carry those words with me while I exercise to this day.

Were you ever afraid you were not doing the exercises correctly?

Yes. I felt nervous and afraid that I would forget how to do my exercises. What helped tremendously was the binder from Beth, filled with pictures and instructions on how to do my exercises.

She also videotaped me performing these exercises and voiced over instructions on how to do them independently; I went home with those videotapes, too.

Whenever I began to question myself, I would either read my binder or watch the video again. This made a world of difference while reinforcing these exercises by myself.

My physical therapist has not created a binder or recorded my exercises. What should I do?

If your physical therapist does not create a binder or video, ask if you can record a portion of the session on your own camera for future reference. I also recommend taking notes and writing down what you learned **immediately** after your physical therapy appointment.

Does your back pain ever come back?

Yes, my back pain comes back when I do not exercise regularly. However, once I go back on my wallboard, the pain dissipates immediately!

How do you stay motivated?

Finding motivation starts within yourself. For me, motivation has always stemmed from maintaining a pain-free life from my scoliosis.

For someone who does not experience pain from their scoliosis, I want you to think of doing your scoliosis-specific exercises as something you are doing to benefit YOUR health! Having the ability to singlehandedly improve your health is such an empowering feeling.

Do you find it harder or easier to exercise regularly today?

Harder. Balancing school and work while budgeting time to exercise is challenging. The key is to maintain a structured schedule that works best for you.

If there is anything that this method of treatment has taught me outside of scoliosis, it's time management.

My physical therapist spends 15 minutes with me, works with other patients, and then rotates back to me at the end. Is that ok?

No, that is NOT okay. If you are being seen by a physical therapist that has been certified by the Barcelona Scoliosis Physical Therapy School, your session should be one-on-one for 45 minutes.

Always Remember...

Your spine's health deserves the same amount of effort you would put into something you feel passionate doing. Whether that passion comes from a sport, playing an instrument, or drawing, please dedicate that same amount of time in taking care of your scoliosis.

PART 3

Parent Support

Imagine you are on an airplane. Shortly before takeoff, you are given instructions to put your oxygen mask on first before you attempt to help others. Likewise, if you are going to help your child manage the turbulence of scoliosis, first and foremost, you need to be properly equipped.

As parents, we have the responsibility for making decisions on behalf of our children and often being their voice. Reading through this section will help validate your experience, while empowering you with information to navigate not just the medical aspects of scoliosis but the psychological and educational arenas as well.

So, put on that oxygen mask and read on!

Signs & Symptoms of Scoliosis

When your child bends forward, does one side of her back appear higher than the other? Is one shoulder elevated? Do you notice any asymmetry? These are some of the physical signs we commonly see, and may overlook:

- Uneven hips, shoulders or waist asymmetry—one side of the waist may be straight and the other more curved
- Rib protrusion when bending forward
- Protruding shoulder blade
- Leg length discrepancy
- Back pain
- Difficulty/discomfort standing for long periods
- Difficulty/discomfort walking for long periods
- Leaning to one side
- Head off-center from trunk
- Uneven creasing of lower back skin
- Uneven breast
- Uneven skirt/dress lengths due to the unevenness in the hips
- Tendency to wear sweatshirts or oversized clothing

Five Stages of Coping with Scoliosis

Some 50 years ago, a Swiss psychiatrist named Elisabeth Kübler-Ross famously described five stages of grief—sometimes known by the acronym DABDA, for denial, anger, bargaining, depression, and acceptance. She introduced the model in her book, On Death and Dying. In the years that followed, the book prompted some debate—mostly because people thought that individuals had to experience all five stages, in a specific order. Kübler-Ross subsequently acknowledged that the stages are not linear, and some people may not experience any of them. Others may experience some stages but not all.

Kübler-Ross' Five Stages of Coping with Grief provides a framework for understanding the process of how children, parents, and families cope with and adapt to scoliosis. What we've sought to do below is to adapt, and build out the psychiatrist's work to help explain the different stages and how they might apply to someone with scoliosis. To be sure, stages of coping are fluid, meaning that not everyone will start at the same place, nor experience all the stages, let alone proceed through them in a linear way. Instead, over the course of time, we may see children and parents exhibit features of all stages.

The five stages in relation to scoliosis are:

Denial

This is the initial reaction we may have when first learning bad news. Pre-teens/teens diagnosed with scoliosis often do not want to acknowledge its existence. Kids who present with denial tend to be ashamed of having scoliosis. They may try to deny the unevenness of their body, avoid treatment, particularly bracing, while minimizing the risks of scoliosis.

Anger

Newly diagnosed children will often wonder, "Why me?" reflecting a sense of injustice as to why this disorder is happening to them. Anger will be displayed in increased arguments with parents over bracing compliance, as well as non-scoliosis issues.

Bargaining

"Let's Make a Deal." Active negotiations may ensue around how long, how often, when and when not they can wear their brace, participate in an exercise regime, or other recommended treatments. The effect of these negotiations is that the responsibility for decision-making falls squarely onto parents. At this stage, often because of a child's bargaining, families may seek out alternative treatments in a desperate attempt to have their child comply with treatment. The risk at this juncture is in being vulnerable to treatments that may not really be helpful and can result in losing precious time to employ more evidence-based approaches.

Depression

When efforts at bargaining prove futile, often after being confronted with curve progression as evidenced by a new set of X-rays and measurements, a feeling of sadness and resignation may start to set in. The child may begin to withdraw and isolate from peer contact and even from activities that they would normally tend to enjoy; they may sometimes appear to be walking around "in a fog." In response to bracing or more appointments for treatment, children in this stage might say, "I'm going to have surgery anyway, so why bother."

Acceptance

This is the stage of coming to terms with a scoliosis diagnosis, as well as recommended treatment(s). In this stage, children accept the reality that they have a condition that makes them different from other children, and which needs to be attended to in a way dictated by physicians and medical practitioners. It is a concession of power, realizing that the innocence of a "normal" body is physically gone and recognizing that this new reality of a spinal curvature with a treatment regimen is the current reality. It does not mean that the child is "okay" with having scoliosis, but they are now accepting of this new reality.

TEEN REACTIONS

Our children will use these various styles of coping when dealing with the challenges of scoliosis and wearing a brace. Some common scenarios and their corresponding coping stages are:

Refusers: (denial, anger, depression) don't want to have anything to do with scoliosis or brace treatment;

Pretenders: (denial, anger, depression) feign compliance, such as wearing the brace to school and then hiding it in their locker;

Negotiators: (denial, anger, bargaining) place the responsibility onto parent(s) of how long, how often, when and when not to wear the brace or exercise; often bargaining with parents;

Hiders: (anger, depression, acceptance) dutifully wear their brace and hope no one notices;

Accepters: (acceptance) compliant with brace wear and all recommended interventions, speak openly about their scoliosis.

Parents will oftentimes reach out to the Curvy Girls' support group when their child is either in the denial or depression stage and they are seeking help to get their child to agree to either follow through with bracing or, at least, feel better about their plight. In contrast, the girls that contact Curvy Girls directly are usually nearing the acceptance stage, but want guidance and affirmation from other girls in navigating the experience of scoliosis. The Curvy Girls' support group experience enhances both acceptance and treatment compliance.

PARENT REACTIONS

And, of course, parents have their own reactions. While some parents are not familiar with the signs and symptoms of scoliosis, once diagnosed, other parents might ignore or minimize their child's scoliosis due to fear of the unknown. Some parents may readily accept the diagnosis of scoliosis and the required regimen of treatment, but minimize any emotional impact it has on their child. Parents may go on "auto pilot," methodically isolating feelings, while concentrating on what needs to be done and not allowing emotions to take control. The "things to do" agenda prevails and dictates the plan for adapting to life with scoliosis.

Parents in the anger stage tend toward self-blame. They feel angry and guilty because this happened to their child under their watch. There's a sense of having failed parental duty, "I'm the parent. My job is to protect my child. Where did I go wrong? Why didn't I see the signs of this sooner?"

Among all the medical appointments and the organizing of files and records, parents eventually get faced with moments that allow for self-reflection and haunting self-doubt. The "what ifs" may consume us. We blame ourselves for not knowing what we could have done differently in order to prevent this from happening to our child. Bargaining with God is not uncommon, as we would gladly commit to performing better in life for a good prognosis for our child. We wish this were happening to us instead of our child. We offer our higher power, or anyone else who will listen, that we would wear the back brace for our child and gladly undergo surgery if it meant sparing them this nightmare.

Depression is a natural and necessary step in the process of healing our grief. After all, it is a sad event in life for a child to be diagnosed with a condition that threatens their health, physical appearance, and psyche. This phase can feel like it will never end and there is a reducing prospect of hope. Watching your child cry and not have a quick fix is quite difficult, but as parents we need to put our personal fears aside and model resilience. Talking about our feelings and getting our thoughts outside of our heads, which happens in the parents' support group at many Curvy Girls' meetings, will provide the first steps toward healing.

In time we all reach acceptance of our new reality. The way we interact with our child, our spouse, other family members, and friends starts to hold a lot less intensity and general tension. Parents can talk a little more freely about their child's scoliosis. Here we can offer our child a respectable, more accomplished role model, one who can offer life examples of how setbacks and challenges are an unavoidable part of life. This, ironically, offers us opportunities to learn critical life skills. Acceptance can help you to segue into a new level of hope and human growth.

How we speak to our children will help them in the process of acceptance. Iyanla Vanzant describes the power of Maya Angelou's words as, "Little energy pellets that shoot forth into the invisible realm of life.

Although we cannot see the words, words become the energy that fills a room, home environment, and our minds."

With this philosophy, the next time you take your child shopping for clothes, instead of saying you'll help her find clothes that *hide* her brace, suggest going shopping for clothes that will best *complement* her brace. Simple changes in our words can have the biggest impact.

Preparing for Your Child's Medical Visit

THINGS TO CONSIDER WHEN CHOOSING AN ORTHOPEDIST:

- Is the orthopedist board certified in orthopedics?
- Do they specialize in scoliosis?
- How many children with scoliosis do they treat each year?
- How many adults with scoliosis do they treat each year?
- Do you know anyone whose child was treated by this physician? How was their care and do they relate well to kids?
- Do they recommend scoliosis-specific exercises as part of the treatment plan?

Parents and children can prepare together for medical visits. Make sure to ask your child what questions they may have. Children may need to be encouraged to ask their questions.

QUESTIONS TO ASK AT THE MEDICAL VISIT(S):

- How many curves?
- What are the curve degrees?
- What are the curve rotations?
- Is calcium and vitamin D3 supplements recommended?
- Which method determines when my child is skeletally mature? (Risser score or Sanders Hand X-ray)
- How often are X-rays taken?

- Is there an EOS imaging nearby?
- If your child has pain, ask: What might be causing the pain?
- Is Physical Therapy Scoliosis Specific Exercises (Schroth, Rigo Method, SEAS) recommended?
- How frequently are follow-up visits scheduled?
- At what curve degree is surgery recommended?
- Where is the closest Curvy Girls' chapter?

Bracing

- How many hours a day is bracing recommended?
- What type of brace is recommended?
- Are all braces equal in terms of effectiveness for preventing curve progression?
- When does brace weaning begin?
- If the brace is to be worn during school hours, request a letter stating diagnosis and accommodations for removing and storing the brace, as well as anything else that will increase bracing compliance during school hours. (See Advocating for Your Child in the School System)

POST VISIT CHECK-IN

Pay attention to what you HEAR, THINK and FEEL as a way to help you process the information and experience. Don't dismiss what you feel, as this is just as valuable as the information you receive.

Conduct a self-check by considering the following:

- What did you **hear**? Remember to write down what you heard.
- What do you **think** about what you heard? Did it create more questions?

- How did the visit make you **feel** overall? How did you feel about the provider, staff and office? Did you feel respected? Heard? Did provider relate to your child?

Check-in with your child to help process their experience. Here there are no right or wrong answers. You are providing a forum for communication between you and your child. Adapt the following prompts based upon your child's developmental stage:

- What did you **hear** ... anything that you didn't understand?
- What do you **think** ... about the doctor you just met?
- How do you **feel** ... about the visit? What did you like about the visit? Was there anything you didn't like?

PUTTING IT ALL TOGETHER

The next challenge is knowing what to do with all the information. How will you keep track and remember?

The answer is simple—keep your records in an electronic device, if you're so inclined, or purchase a notebook/binder with built-in folders. Separate the sections: Surgeons, Orthotist, Physical Therapist, Psychologist and even Curvy Girls.

Bring your notebook/binder to all your appointments to jot down what was discussed. For example, if you saw your child's surgeon, your notes might include:

- Today's date
- Curve degree(s)
- Date diagnosed
- Type of curve(s)
- Number out-of-brace hours prior to X-ray
- X-rays (Yes/No)
- Exam results (no change, increase, decrease)
- Recommend scoliosis specific exercises
- Gave a Curvy Girls' flyer for support group meetings
- Follow-up visit (every 4–6 months)

Prior to leaving, take five minutes and finish writing all the information you heard while it is still fresh in your mind. These new habits will ultimately leave you feeling less stressed and more in control of your child's care.

To learn more tips on how to maintain your child's medical information, visit: PulseCenterForPatientSafety.org.

What If Your Child Needs Surgery?

You've just found out your child needs spinal fusion surgery and your anxiety level is through the roof. Just reading that statement is enough to send shivers down our spines.

As uncomfortable as anxiety can feel, it serves a purpose in our lives, alerting us to an event filled with unknowns. Anxiety can immobilize us or if used as intended, propel us into motion. Ask yourself what exactly are you anxious about? Are your fears based in reality or not?

GET THE FACTS!

Gather information from trusted sources—medical providers, informed families, reading materials.

Get your thoughts out of your head—write down exactly what you are afraid of and speak them aloud to a trusted person. Learning what to expect from your child's surgery puts you at an advantage. Ask questions and gather information. If your child says they are worried, anxious or concerned, ask them to write down their worries. Help them get the facts.

Learn what is a rational (reality) worry versus a worry that is not based in reality (irrational). When we don't understand something that we're anxious about, we fill in the blanks with our own scary thoughts. Don't leave empty spaces. Fill in the blanks with facts. Knowledge is power.

PEOPLE HANDLE FEAR DIFFERENTLY

Some people cope better with more information, while others would rather not have details of the operation and prefer to leave it up to the expert. Know and respect your own and your child's coping style.

Would your child like to ask more questions and find out more detail about the surgery or would she prefer to not participate in this conversation. A general rule of thumb is the younger the child, the less details they are interested in. However, some older teens may want to ask more questions and should be afforded that opportunity.

Some of our girls reach out for tools prior to surgery, others cope by pushing surgery out of their mind until the night before. Whatever their method, honor it.

It is particularly important that we not impose our reactions/feelings onto our child. Kids look to their adults to find out what is normal. If you are confident and positive, generally your child will follow suit. If you are anxious and worried, your child may become more anxious and worried or possibly deny their own feelings in order not to worry you. Your child will have their own feelings, concerns, and worries and do not need to take on yours.

LOCATE A SUPPORT GROUP

The sinking feeling in the pit of your stomach can be eased when meeting post-surgery moms smiling and speaking confidently about their daughter's surgery and recovery. After all, would they be smiling if it were that awful? Happy post-surgery moms help to normalize a situation filled with unknowns.

Seek out a local Curvy Girls' support group where you can speak with other parents who are dealing with the same issues. If there isn't a support group in your area, consider online support. The difficulty sometimes with seeking support through social media is reading unfiltered accounts of others' stories without having all the facts. This could potentially create additional worries.

Get the facts, know your coping style, trust the pilot and remember to breathe. I'm smiling and soon you will be too!

Never worry alone!

Make a plan!

And remember, keep things in proper perspective!

KEEP IN MIND

The thought of your child undergoing spine surgery is frightening, yet remembering that it's part of your surgeon's normal day can be most helpful.

Are you good at your job or things you like to do? Do you perform certain tasks over and over until they become second nature? Thinking about surgery is overwhelming, in part because it is not something for which we have any familiarity.

A thought that Robin found reassuring while leading up to and especially during the hours of Leah's surgery was "While this day is anything but normal to us, it is a typical work day for our surgeon—nothing extraordinary or unusual." In fact, scoliosis surgery is actually fairly straightforward, neither exploratory or diagnostic. This mindset is what she now shares with anxious parents whose child is awaiting surgery.

Try to hold onto that thought if you find it reassuring.

Just another day of doing what they do best!

PLANNING THE HOSPITAL STAY

Contact the hospital to find out what is provided and what you'll need to bring, e.g., extra blanket, pillow. Sometimes hospitals permit or invite you to tour the setting. The more you normalize an experience, the less scary it is. Visit the hospital if permitted so you and your child can become familiar with the surroundings. If your hospital provides a tour, ask your child if she'd like to go. Speaking with staff at the hospital can be very reassuring and allay some anxiety.

Inquire about a Child Life Specialist whose purpose is to help minimize the stress of being in a hospital setting. They can make your child's hospital stay more pleasant with activities, while providing on-site emotional support for both you and your child.

- **Promote scar healing** with a product orthopedic surgeon Dr. James Barsi recommends, Dermabond Prineo® applied at the end of surgery. You can ask your surgeon if they are willing to use this product too.

- **Wash, condition, and braid hair** the night before surgery. Ohio Curvy Mom Sandy Dorton says, "If African American, do not pay a Braider a lot of money to have this done before surgery. In case they do neurotesting with head electrodes, the hospital will probably make you take them down. Check with the hospital to be sure."

- **Pack simply** and don't overpack. We do not suggest buying new undergarments, pajamas or robe. In addition to the likelihood of them getting ruined, they are generally too restrictive following a scoliosis surgery. Hospital gowns are the best options because they provide ease for getting in and out of, as well as ease of access for medical staff. Simply double-up on hospital gowns with the second one used as a bathrobe to cover their back.

Your child will need non-skid slip-on shoes or slippers. Soft headbands may be helpful to keep loose hair off face. Your child will also not need much to keep them occupied, as they will not have the ability to stay focused for any length of time.

For parents, wear and bring comfortable clothing and slip-on shoes with sweater/sweatshirt and yoga pants for sleeping.

Items that Curvy Girls' parents find helpful:

- Toiletries: toothbrush, toothpaste, dry shampoo, lip balm/chapstick, face wipes

- Electronics: tablet or laptop, phone, with chargers and headphones

- Magazines, book, craft to keep parent occupied while daughter rests/sleeps

- Reading light or phone flashlight as an alternative to bright overhead lights

- Water bottles, healthy snacks, sugarless gum, lozenges

- Notebook with related paperwork

- Prescription medications

- Face mask that can be chilled for swollen eyes after surgery

DAY OF SURGERY

Once signed in at hospital, you and your child will be brought to pre-op. In some hospitals this is the same area as post-op. Here your child will exchange her clothing for a hospital gown. Consider asking the attending nurse to leave on your child's panties until after she is sedated, which will leave your child feeling less exposed, especially if menstruating.

Ohio Curvy Mom Sandy Dorton advises: "Surgery can last up to six + hours so take books, phone charger, puzzles, snacks and a support person who doesn't make you crazy."

"Plan on spending the night; I stayed at night and my husband came in the morning to relieve me. I didn't get much sleep with nurses coming in to check on my daughter Alyse."

HOSPITAL STAY

- **Treat everyone with respect** "from the person who empties the trash in your room to the doctor who performs the surgery. If you do, you will be treated the same way," advises New Jersey Curvy Mom Patty Borzner.

- **Be your child's advocate** and don't be afraid to speak up on your child's behalf. Insist that everyone who enters the hospital room is healthy and sanitizes their hands upon arrival. The last thing you or your child need is to get a cold or cough on top of everything else you're dealing with.

- **Help manage your child's pain.** A pain medicine pump (PCA) should be arranged with your surgeon in advance. This allows your child to control their medication in response to pain. Pain needs to be managed. Leah, for example, never had to experience pain beyond what she could tolerate. "That's what pain medications are for," said Beth Roach, pediatric intensive care nurse. "Allowing the patient to 'bear the pain' is actually counterproductive and can prolong healing time. In order to heal, patients need to breathe deeply and move frequently, neither of which they can do while in pain."

- **Walking post-surgery** is recommended by John Denneen, physical therapist and administrator for Hospital of Special Surgery. "Walk first thing the next morning after surgery. Walk before fear sets in."

  Sitting upright and moving is highly recommended by medical professionals to help with the healing process, resulting in a quicker recovery and return home. Do NOT allow your child to lay in bed for extended periods of time and certainly not the whole day. Not all hospitals have the staffing to stay on top of your child's activity level, so you may need to take the lead.

- **Chew sugarless gum** following surgery, advises Pediatric Rehab physical therapist Marissa Muccio, in order to help with gas/bloating and moving bowels. Citing a small study, she recommends "chewing sugarless gum five times per day for 20 minutes after surgery to speed up the first bowel movement, a critical part of hospital discharge/comfort."

- **Stay hydrated** by drinking plenty of fluids, especially water to avoid constipation.

- **Constipation** can occur from anesthesia, pain medication, lack of food and water. It's a good idea to have a bowel movement sometime before leaving the hospital, to avoid dealing with constipation at home. For constipation, increase fiber and water intake and discuss medication for use at home with medical staff.

GOING HOME

- **Bring plenty of pillows** for ride home, suggests Long Island Curvy Mom, Regina Papile.

- **Drive least bumpy route** to minimize discomfort from jolting

- **Review discharge instructions** before leaving the hospital. Make sure you have a clear understanding and that all questions have been answered. Confirm that all prescriptions for home have been sent to your local pharmacy. While at home don't be afraid to call the hospital staff with any questions.

- **Wear comfortable clothing** such as a button-down shirt with loose fitting sweatpants for exiting the hospital. Wearing a bra post-surgery is difficult. After a couple weeks once scar is healed, bralette, bandeaus or soft sports bras are recommended.

AT HOME

- **Body pillow** to add more comfort while resting or sleeping

- **Heating pad or gel packs** may be soothing. Ask your doctor when these would be appropriate to use.

- **Avoid recliners or soft chairs**, as they tend to be difficult to rise from, advises Long Island Curvy Mom Debbie Zenz, whose daughter, Danielle, got stuck in one for more than an hour. You will want to make sure that she has access to a firm chair with arms she can use to help her stand.

- **Slip-on shoes** rather than ones with laces. Bending down is difficult, and that includes bending down to tie shoes.
- **Go slow getting up from bed.** Start by setting up the bed far enough away from the wall so that you can walk on both sides. That way, a parent or caregiver can lend a hand. Mom Debbie says, "I bent down so Danielle could hold onto my shoulders as I stood up. In this way, she was using my leverage to stand."
- **Consider using hospital-type "chuck pads"** to ease movement to the edge of the bed. The plastic on the bottom of a chuck pad moves easily across the sheets, allowing you to pull your child towards you without much effort on her part, or yours. Another idea might be satin sheets for easy sliding.
- **Think about having a bed on the first floor** for less stair-climbing and staying closer to the action. Since Leah's room was upstairs, her parents opted to temporarily set up a hospital bed on the first floor. That meant Leah wouldn't have to worry about climbing stairs and she would be closer to family members during the day.
- **A hospital bed can make things easier** but isn't necessary. The hospital bed's incline and side rails helped Leah to be more self-reliant when getting up. Her mom, Robin, slept on the couch next to her just in case anything was needed in the middle of the night. Insurance companies will pay for a temporary hospital bed if prescribed by your surgeon.
- **Showering** is not permitted until you get clearance from your surgeon. However, with a shower chair, salon cape, and hand-held shower sprayer you can wash your child's hair when she feels up to it.

    Robin's nurse neighbor suggested using a light-weight aluminum lawn chair rather than a surgical seat for her daughter Leah's showers. The lawn chair proved less cumbersome than a medical shower chair. Remember, the incision can't get wet until all the bandages, known as Steri-Strips™, fall off. While a salon cape is an option, Robin used a large plastic garbage bag and put a hole in the bottom for Leah's hair and head to come out and be washed—like the Caped Crusader on a Lawn Chair!

Note that a hospital chair is considerably sturdier, so this should be taken into consideration when making a decision.

- **Carefully read and follow the instructions for all pain medications.** Surgical patients will go home with a prescription for oral pain medication. Robin realized too late that she had been giving Leah the same amount of medication that she had been getting in the hospital—twice as much as the surgeon had prescribed for home. It was only when Leah started running out of pain medication that her mother read the instructions and realized her mistake. It's very important to create a medication chart and journal the times each medication is given.
- **Optional items**—foam top mattress, raised toilet seat with handles, hand-held shower head, hospital bed.

Parents say that the weeks post-surgery in many ways may come to feel like when you took care of your child as a baby—on-call and exhausted. Your adolescent child who fought for independence will now become totally dependent upon you, but temporarily.

We know you will worry about your child but remember with youth on their side, they bounce back very quickly. Similar to what you've heard or experienced with childbirth, once over, it will become a faded memory with a healthy child on the other side.

Advocating for Your Child in The School System

Ellen Stoltz, PhD

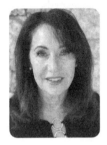

Ellen Stoltz, PhD *is an educational consultant certified in Pre-K through Grade 12 general and special education; she holds a doctorate in education.*

As a special education teacher and Senior Director of Students Support Services in the Hartford Public Schools, Dr. Stoltz focused on ensuring students with diverse learning needs, Individualized Education Programs (IEPs) and Section 504 Plans could access and benefit from all aspects of general education. Dr. Stoltz contributed significantly to educational improvements in the Bloomfield Public Schools in her role as Chief Academic Officer. With the personal approach to accommodations found in Section 504 Plans and IEPs, Dr. Stoltz ensured that every student had the tools to succeed in the general education setting.

UNDERSTANDING AND UTILIZING SECTION 504 PLANS

Your school is the perfect environment to teach your child how to become an independent thinker and doer. The general education classroom is a microcosm of your local culture, where advocating for oneself is paramount to success academically, socially and emotionally. What an opportune situation for your child with scoliosis to practice what you model and encourage as a parent!

United States Federal Law, Section 504 of the Americans with Disabilities Act (ADA), protects the rights of pre-kindergarten through grade 12 students with any medical condition that affects their quality of learning in the general education environment. As a civil rights statute, your child diagnosed with scoliosis is entitled to school accommodations under this law.

The process of developing and implementing effective, realistic Section 504 Plans can contribute to your child's sense of independence. The plan, of course, begins with what your child wants and needs to succeed in school relative to the effects of scoliosis in the school setting. A direct conversation chockful of listening and learning on your part to what your child wants should happen at every age through young adulthood. Your child will understand your perspective for advocacy with increasing meaningfulness at different developmental stages. Most children with scoliosis require similar accommodations, often attributed to the physical effects and discomfort of wearing a brace or having had surgery.

Here are some of the items that have been included in Section 504 Plans for students with scoliosis:

- Extra time as needed for the following scenarios:
  - Leaving class three minutes early in order to avoid being pushed; maneuvering in a back brace can be difficult. Rushing through halls or stairwells can be potentially harmful for a child wearing a back brace
  - Accessing locker prior to next class, if needed
  - Allot designated amount of time for changing in pre-designated private area, such as the school nurse's bathroom, prior to and following physical education classes
- Pre-approval pass for nurse visits, as needed
- Extra set of textbooks at home, E-books from publishers
- Ensure opportunity to move around (or even leave) classrooms or hallways
- Adjust chair and table height for sitting or standing as needed
- Assign locker with height suitable to your child to eliminate the need for bending
- Provide a safe place to store brace when not being worn
- Ensure your child is exempt from active participation in bus drills (Your child should not be jumping out of the bus wearing a back brace)
- For tornado drills, your child should squat instead of bending
- Provide daily elevator pass or personal key, if stairs are a problem

- Physical Education activity should be modified based on what the child is able to do and should avoid (see page 231)

- Provide air conditioner or fan in an overheated classroom as needed to help a braced child tolerate the heat (Inform the 504 Team members that back braces do not allow air flow and your child can easily become overheated.)

- Arrange school bus transportation pickup close to or in front of your home

Accommodations specific to your child's school building and physical needs should always be discussed with input from your child and school-based staff. Every school building has a unique configuration, with physical features that may not be readily apparent until they become problematic for your child.

Your child may require specific accommodations particular to bracing, scoliosis curvature, pre- and post-surgery, and the school's physical environment. This may require more intensive advocacy on your part in activating your child's voice as a call for action and support.

Specifically, the steps in advocating include identifying the problem and the people who can support solutions, strategizing ideas, negotiating realistic solutions, and developing, implementing and adjusting the plan.

Here are ten strategies to ensure the Section 504 Plan addresses your child's needs from elementary school to college:

1. Review and summarize needs and wants with your child before every meeting.

2. List what is working and what is not (needs and wants), shifting more responsibility each year to your child to complete.

3. Encourage your child to present at least one item from the list to the Section 504 Planning Team. Over time, this will help them to learn how to advocate for themselves.

4. Find common ground with school-based staff and be prepared to negotiate!

5. Ensure the school identifies a Case Manager and communication mode (email, text) to facilitate ongoing communication.

6. Request distribution of 504 Plan to your child's teachers.

7. Check in periodically with Case Manager for positives and challenges.

8. Request a Transition meeting between grade levels and building changes.

9. Shift ownership of problem-solving and advocacy to your child by saying "That's a big problem...How would you like to address this?" For high school and college students, you might ask, "How are you planning to solve it?"

    There are many ways to spark independent thinking in your child. Find the vocabulary or dialogue that works for you AND your child and stick with it.

10. Give specific positive feedback to your child for speaking up by saying "You identified what you needed, asked for help and solved the problem!"

Please be aware that private schools and universities are exempt from the requirements of Section 504, as these schools typically do not receive federal funding. Private colleges and universities are required to address reasonable accommodations through the Americans with Disabilities Act (ADA).

Keeping a successful school, college and career experience in mind as the goal for your child, these tips can guide you as you and your child uncover gaps and respond proactively to address challenges. In this manner, you can demonstrate to your child concrete ways to develop his/her own voice and navigate solutions to provide the accommodations to which he/she is entitled.

PART 4

Understanding the World of Bracing

When our girls were initially diagnosed, we were not aware of bracing options other than the one recommended by our surgeon. We simply took the doctor's script and often chose the closest orthotist to our home.

This section is intended to help educate and guide you while navigating the world of scoliosis bracing. Designed to find information quickly, we've organized this section into a series of questions and answers that can be used as a resource when choosing both an orthotist and brace type.

We hope that the viewpoints from these orthotists will help you to make the best decision for your child.

Please note that the responses reflect each professional's experiences, perceptions, and beliefs about bracing. Since each curve and patient's circumstances are unique, it is important to consult your child's entire scoliosis treatment team—orthopedist, physical therapist and orthotist—with any questions.

Michael Mangino CPO, CPed, LPO

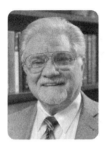

Michael Mangino, *founder and operator of Bay Orthopedics on Long Island (bayorthopedic.com), is both a licensed and American Board Certified Orthotist and Prosthetist and Board Certified Pedorthist. He holds several patents in the Orthotics and Sports Medicine field. His research has been published and he has been interviewed by various journals within the profession. He has served the profession as a founder and Board member of the New York Orthotics and Prosthetics Association and instructor to several of New York's universities.*

What is an Orthotist?

An orthotist is a healthcare professional who provides care to patients with disabling conditions of the spine and limbs, by fitting and fabricating orthopedic devices (orthoses) under the direction and in consultation with physicians.

How do you select a qualified Orthotist?

Your orthopedist will provide you with the name(s) of orthotist(s). You may also want to check with other parents for their recommendations. It is important that an orthotist be board-certified in orthotics, and that they received additional post-graduate training in the use of scoliotic bracing. It is also beneficial for your orthotist to be trained in the use of several different types of scoliosis devices.

From your experience, how important is the orthotist-patient relationship?

In addition to finding a qualified orthotist, it is important to ensure that the orthotist be able to establish a rapport with you and your child. Because brace compliance is a big issue with teen bracing, teens need to feel comfortable with their orthotist, and have trust in what they are saying. The orthotist needs to be able to hear and respond to your child's concerns in order to increase the likelihood of compliance. Your child will not wear their brace if it hurts. Orthotists should make themselves available to both parent and child for questions or problems related to bracing.

Why does a child need to wear a brace?

The purpose of bracing children with scoliosis is to stabilize the curve from progressing until the patient is finished growing in height. Conventional TLSO Bracing is not intended to reduce or correct scoliosis curves. HOWEVER... three- and four-dimensional bracing has demonstrated that curves can be reduced significantly.

What should a new patient anticipate when initially wearing their first brace?

- A properly fitting scoliosis brace is snug.
- Bracing may be uncomfortable, but it should NOT hurt.
- There may be redness where the brace applies pressure. However, redness that does not clear in fifteen minutes after removing the brace, as well as sores or blisters, are immediate signs to contact your orthotist for a brace adjustment.
- Bracing should begin with a few hours a day, gradually increasing over several days until the recommended hours are reached.

Important: If pain is caused by the brace, return to the orthotist to determine the source of the discomfort. The pain should always be able to be relieved. **Irritation and pain caused by the brace is unacceptable.**

What kind of correction should be expected from the first in-brace X-ray?

Traditionally, the aim is to achieve a 50% reduction of curves for the first in-brace X-ray.

That statement was probably accurate when referring to a TLSO style brace, such as the Boston Brace. However, when utilizing the concepts of three-dimensional bracing, the emphasis is on designing a derotation, corrective brace that allows us to achieve a 30° to 70° correction for the first in-brace X-ray. With that being said, the amount of correction is also contingent on the flexibility of the spine and bone age of the patient.

For many years you fabricated one type of TLSO brace. What changed your way of thinking that there could be a better approach?

In 2012, I attended the first International Curvy Girls Scoliosis Convention where I met Grant Wood and was introduced to three-dimensional bracing. During that same conference, I also attended a presentation on the Schroth Method and learned that by working on reducing rotation through 3D bracing in conjunction with scoliosis-specific exercises, you could possibly reverse the scoliotic curvatures. After the conference, I decided to educate myself further on both of these concepts and have now dedicated my practice to educating both orthopedic surgeons and newly diagnosed families about these two viable treatment options.

The primary objective of bracing is to stop a curve from progressing. Over the years how much has changed in the way you view that statement?

To be honest, it changed quite a bit. In the United States, most orthotists were taught that scoliosis bracing was only capable of stopping a curve from progressing. However, after going through the extensive training process of the Rigo Chêneau three-dimensional bracing, I can now state that in almost 50% of our cases we have been able to reverse the scoliosis curves by the time their bracing journey is complete. That's a bold statement, but accurate and now realistic to achieve.

Can all 3D bracing accomplish this?

No. Just because a brace is marketed as 3-dimensional does not mean it's corrective or a Rigo Chêneau brace. When you are stating 3-dimensional, it means you are attempting to affect the rotational component of scoliosis that affects all three planes of the body—coronal, sagittal and axial. Unfortunately, not all 3D braces that are being fabricated are accomplishing that objective.

How is the training different when learning 3-dimensional bracing?

Learning this corrective technique using a WCR (Wood Chêneau Rigo) brace took two intensive years of training, in addition to being a Board Certified Orthotist. This specific bracing concept is very challenging because you are studying the body in the transverse plane while learning how to classify the nine basic Rigo configurations, and then all of the hybrids. And keep in mind, this is a completely different technique than what most orthotist are taught in the United States on brace fitting.

This method of bracing requires many follow-up visits and coordination of care within the scoliosis healthcare team. These teams consist of an orthopedist, orthotist and the physical therapist trained in scoliosis-specific exercises, such as a Schroth therapist.

Are you now able to stabilize more challenging curves using the 3-dimensional approach?

I can honestly state that I now have taken on more difficult curves that were once considered to be within surgical range and reduce them to a point below surgical necessity.

Have you seen curves not only stabilize but reverse from this type of bracing?

With the utilization of true Rigo Chêneau braces, it is common for orthotists to see a reversal of scoliotic curves. That is why they are considered corrective by design. At a recent Society on Scoliosis Orthopedic and Rehabilitation Treatment (SOSORT) convention, a study was presented showing that the average correction was slightly more than ten degrees from patients who were skeletally mature and out of the brace after successfully completing a brace program, as compared to when they first started brace wear. It was even more effective when the patient was also compliant with their Schroth physical therapy.

What curves are most difficult to stabilize?

With conventional TLSO scoliosis bracing, it was virtually impossible to treat a curve with an apex of T6 or higher because the patient's own arm gets in the way. However, a Rigo Chêneau scoliosis brace utilizing a D-modifier technique makes it possible to treat upper thoracic curves as high as T-4.

Are 3-dimensional braces covered by medical insurance?

For many reasons, obtaining coverage of a three-dimensional brace is difficult. In 2004, when Rigo Chêneau braces were introduced into the United States, they were **true** three-dimensional braces and were corrective braces. However, with the increased demand from parents for this kind of brace, many brace manufacturers jumped on the words "3D" and three-dimensional in their brace design although they weren't actually fabricating corrective braces such as Rigo Chêneau braces. As a result, insurance carriers have become confused into thinking that all "labeled" 3D braces are equal when in reality they are not by a long shot.

Additionally, insurance companies like to keep things simple and work in a black and white world where they can limit their liability. They want to provide the most cost-effective brace (least costly) to treat a patient. Therefore, many are satisfied to approve a brace that will **try** to prevent the curve from progressing, while a "true/corrective" brace such as Wood Chêneau Rigo is not only trying to stabilize the curves but also has the ability to **reduce** the scoliosis imbalance and achieve a more cosmetically balanced spine.

The bottom line is that three-dimensional bracing challenges the insurance companies to think about the scoliosis case that they are being asked to approve. Parents and brace providers need to be very clear of this distinction when advocating with insurers. Needless to say, it is a complicated brace that can be described with multiple codes and unique variations of those codes that require substantial documentation. In order to secure optimum or full coverage for our families, we heavily document the case before submitting to the insurance carrier.

What last piece of advice would you give to a new parent about bracing?

- Be your child's advocate.
- Never dismiss the importance of bracing.
- Remember to have your child follow a gradual course of bracing over several days.
- Brace adjustments should relieve any pain.
- Irritations and back pain caused by the brace is unacceptable.
- Never allow a healthcare professional to intimidate you!

Part 4: Understanding the World of Bracing

Luke Stikeleather CO

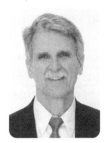

*As a certified orthotist specializing in scoliosis and spinal bracing for more than 30 years, **Luke Stikeleather** is passionate about patient care, developing new treatment concepts and mentoring the next generation of scoliosis practitioners. He is a coauthor on several publications and has given numerous presentations nationally and internationally. He was President of the International Society on Scoliosis Rehabilitation and Treatment, SOSORT, 2018-2019 and has been on the Board of Directors since 2012. He is a member of the Scoliosis Research Society, and is the Founder and President of the National Scoliosis Center in Fairfax, Virginia (nationalscoliosiscenter.com).*

What does the National Scoliosis Center offer to newly diagnosed families?

The National Scoliosis Center [NSC] is one of the first comprehensive treatment centers specializing in the non-operative treatment of scoliosis. Our facility is rather unique in that we employ former patients and parents of patients who can personally relate to the families we treat and are committed to creating pleasant experiences and positive outcomes.

Many newly diagnosed families are anxious or concerned, so we make it a priority to reassure them that we will competently answer all their questions and help them navigate their scoliosis journey. Our thorough patient assessment, X-ray review and detailed education process makes our families comfortable and empowers them to make informed decisions regarding their treatment.

All our braces are fabricated on-site using state-of-the-art 3D shape capture CAD/CAM technology and many of our patients help make their brace. This, along with our EOS low-dose X-ray system, Diers Formetric topographical scanner, and certified Schroth Physical Therapy services, contributes to our reputation as a premier center of excellence.

What advice would you give a new parent when choosing an orthotist and a brace for their child?

A parent's priority is to educate themselves so they can advocate for their child. Find out about "best practice" methods and recommendations. Connect with informed parents and professionals and use resources like Curvy Girls to gain basic knowledge and understanding of the diagnosis and treatment. Make every effort to select the best scoliosis bracing **specialist** available, someone with impeccable reputation and extensive experience, regardless of travel distance and, when possible, regardless of insurance.

Recognize that the average orthotist is a **generalist** who treats a wide range of individuals and conditions; few of them have specific depth or breadth of knowledge, experience, or skill in making scoliosis braces and managing this condition. By all means, parents should seek an orthotist that is not only knowledgeable but someone who is passionate about treating scoliosis patients. Some valuable questions to ask are:

- What specific/specialized scoliosis training have you had?
- Where were you trained and by whom?
- How many years have you been treating scoliosis?
- How many braces do you make each month?
- What brace design do you use?
- What percentage of your work is dedicated to scoliosis versus other orthotic/prosthetic services?

We strongly advocate that doctors, orthotists, therapists, patients and parents study and follow *2016 SOSORT guidelines: orthopaedic and rehabilitation treatment of idiopathic scoliosis during growth,* found online.

Can you give us a background history of the Rigo-Chêneau-type brace and your involvement to bringing it to North America?

The Chêneau Brace originated with French brace developer Dr. Jacques Chêneau. In the 1970s, Dr. Chêneau worked closely with Katharina Schroth and Christa Lehnert-Schroth in Germany incorporating their breathing concepts and curve classifications for scoliosis and physical therapy treatment into his brace designs. Dr. Manuel Rigo of Spain expanded on Dr. Chêneau's work, refining the curve classifications and developing more specific brace designs. Through my time with Dr. Rigo, I started using these principles in the United States in 2004, working closely with Beth Janssen PT, Cindy Marti PT, Amy Sbihli, DPT and others of the first Schroth therapists trained by Dr. Rigo. Our collective success was exciting and over time our work ignited interest from others.

I consider myself a life-long learner, continuously pursuing knowledge and education in order to serve our patients better. My friendship with Dr. Rigo, and involvement with many of my colleagues from SOSORT over the past 17 years, not only enables me to stay current with the principles of scoliosis and the mechanics of bracing, but to be an active innovator in the field. We are mentoring orthotists around the country, helping them to implement 3D bracing in their practice and become true scoliosis specialists.

The Schroth Method encourages a Chêneau TLSO with Rigo modifications. Why does this type of bracing work best for this exercise method?

As previously mentioned, the Schroth Method emphasized specific breathing and movement exercises tailored to each curve pattern, which Dr. Chêneau incorporated in his brace design that had contact points and relief/expansion areas. In current terms, I refer to this as "selective contact" where the brace applies a directional force to move the curvature towards an expansion area opposite the curve. This intentional space allows the spine and torso to move more freely in the desired "corrected" position. Daily movement, breathing, and gradual growth inside the 3D brace create remodeling over time. Despite what some well-intentioned doctors and orthotists say, most traditional braces are "total contact," touching the body all over, blocking the torso from translating and derotating which undermines the effectiveness of the brace and the Schroth therapy. Conversely, the Rigo classification of curve patterns and his corresponding brace design works synergistically with the Schroth approach.

You have been using the principles of 3D bracing for over 30 years. What led you to pursue this type of approach in brace design?

Flat Stanley is a children's book that I read to my girls when they were young. In the fictional story, a chalkboard falls on Stanley making him two dimensional. Stanley has height and width, but no thickness. Similarly, X-rays are 2-dimensional which only gives a view of scoliosis from the front or back. Historically, many 2D brace designs have been constructed to achieve maximum correction of the 2D X-ray. Doctors and orthotists have placed an over-emphasis on reducing the curve(s) by 50% while ignoring the importance of overall body alignment and appearance.

After meeting Dr. Rigo, Dr. Chêneau and others at a Spine Deformities Conference in Barcelona in 2004, I decided to devote the remainder of my career to exclusively serving people with scoliosis and spinal deformities by becoming a spine-scoliosis specialist. Once you understand the basic 3D biomechanical principles of scoliosis, you can never be content with typical 2D braces.

What is distinct about your 3D brace?

Successful scoliosis treatment is like solving a good jigsaw puzzle. You need to identify and properly assemble all the right pieces to complete the big picture.

In my opinion, it is who we are and what we do at NSC that makes our service, not our brace, so distinctive. Although we are strong advocates for designing and delivering exceptional 3D braces that fit well and function optimally, we think there is frequently an overemphasis placed on the product, "the brace," with an under-appreciation of the practitioner, purpose, passion, process and protocol.

I draw deeply from my early training as a social worker and family counselor recognizing the importance of seeing and valuing the whole person while addressing their physical scoliosis condition. We provide each patient with an individualized, specific treatment plan. We have a proven strategy of engaging each person in the process of their care. Developed with the treatment team, our protocol provides clear directives for proper brace wear, time in brace, regular brace rechecks and X-rays to be followed for the course of treatment.

What kind of success have you had with this method of bracing?

Since switching to the Rigo-Chêneau type brace in 2004, I have made over five thousand braces. By our calculation, 90% of our patients have had successful results—meaning no surgery was needed. Of that 90%, 60% of patients saw curve stabilization—an important outcome considering the progressive nature of scoliosis, especially during the adolescent years. Surprisingly, 30% experienced curve improvement. The remaining 10%, referred to as bracing failures, most often progressed due to large magnitude curves at initial treatment (3%) or patient non-compliance (7%).

What do you attribute the success to?

We know that brace compliance and a successful outcome requires complete "buy in" from the patient and their parents! In addition to providing a well-designed, properly fit brace, it is essential to address the mind and heart of the patient while also treating their body. This process starts with educating them with knowledge about scoliosis and explaining why they need a brace, what wearing a brace will be like, and what the brace is doing for their condition. Our staff, many of whom are former patients or parents of patients, share their own personal experiences and we often have new girls meet current patients in the office. We also encourage them to connect with others in the local Curvy Girls' group. This helps put them at ease and prepares them for the journey that lies ahead.

We view our role as a "scoliosis safari guide" who expertly and safely helps our patients navigate their challenging journey. Our constant presence and support throughout their journey leads to improved compliance and outcomes. Our team employs many strategies to enhance the "human factor" of the treatment plan. Frequent follow-up visits, brace checks, and adjustments allow for opportunities to provide feedback, encouragement, and motivation. Accountability is important, so we occasionally use monitoring devices to check true wearing time. Our positive attitudes can be infectious and inspiring. We know that a patient's positive attitude is the key ingredient to their success.

Can you describe a challenging correction you were able to achieve as a result of your three-dimensional approach to bracing?

We have many of these, but I will highlight one. Lexi came to us from Canada with two large curves approaching 50° at first diagnosis. The doctor was doubtful that a brace would be of any benefit, but he was willing to provide the paperwork and opportunity to attempt bracing. Not wanting surgery, Lexi was very motivated to wear a brace. Desperate for competent care, her family found us through our website. We saw Lexi at 8 a.m., fit her brace that afternoon, made final adjustments the next day, and took an EOS X-ray to confirm that appropriate correction was achieved. We were hopeful that her determination and discipline could prevent curve progression and surgery. Surprisingly, year by year, from age 13 to 16, Lexi's diligence doing Schroth exercise and wearing her brace paid off with improved curve magnitudes. Two years after weaning from the brace, her curves are now below 20°. We have several other similar examples and while **this is not the norm**, it is a positive testimony of what is possible when our protocol is faithfully followed.

At the Scoliosis Research Society conference in 2018, recognition was given to Dr. Negrini, Dr. Donzelli, Dr. Felice, and Dr. Zaina for their presentation "Brace wearing time is strongest predictor of final results." Can you share what this study concluded?

This same team of authors published a follow-up study in July 2018 titled *"Consistent and Regular Wearing Improved Bracing Results: A Case Controlled Study."* The essence of both presentations conclusively demonstrates that more favorable outcomes of curve stabilization or improvement are achieved by patients that consistently wear their braces 22-24 hours per day.

Their research findings validate our own experience and must be continuously emphasized and impressed upon every physician, patient, parent, and practitioner involved in treating scoliosis. The amount of daily wearing time is critical to achieving optimal outcomes!

Is wearing a brace for patients with larger curves, 45°–55°, more uncomfortable?

Brace comfort has more to do with the brace design and the orthotist's skill rather than it does with the curve magnitude. Additionally, our experience enables us to identify different sensitivity levels among patients in order to appropriately treat them. Some patients are tough as nails and can tolerate the brace with few discomfort issues, while others are at the opposite end of the spectrum feeling everything intensely, regardless of the curve size. It is important to understand the patient and demonstrate patience in order to help the patient obtain necessary correction while still being comfortable. The brace may seem strange at first (to all patients), but they should all adapt to the fit and feel with help from their orthotist.

Can excess body weight impact brace correction?

It certainly makes the bracing process more challenging. Braces work by applying pressure to the spine via the ribs and soft tissues. Some research studies have reported that excess body weight/high BMI makes bracing difficult and can negatively impact outcomes. A properly fit brace is still recommended over not wearing a brace at all. Weight should not be a deterrent and a competent scoliosis orthotist should be able to construct a well fit brace. Morbid obesity comes with its own unique set of challenges for a patient. Not only is the patient's overall health at risk, but so is the health of the spine and skeleton. It is always important to consider the whole patient when creating a treatment plan.

Does bracing address hyperkyphosis and hyperlordosis?

Ideally, every human spine should have some kyphosis and lordosis. These are the normal front to back curves seen when looking at our spine from the side (sagittal view). Excessive curvature called hyperkyphosis and hyperlordosis can be a source of pain and permanent change of alignment or appearance if not effectively treated with bracing and physical therapy in a timely manner. Gradual growth-guided correction can be achieved when a properly designed and fit brace is diligently worn at least 21-23 hours per day until skeletal maturity is complete.

It is important to mention another sagittal plane condition commonly occurring with scoliosis which is sometimes created or aggravated by poor bracing—hypokyphosis or 'flatback.' This can occur when there is reduced or insufficient kyphosis/lordosis and frequently complicates proper bracing. Too few doctors and orthotists recognize this for the significant problem that it creates to effective bracing and long-term spine health.

Can a 3D brace be effective in preventing progression for skeletally mature young adults with scoliosis?

It is generally accepted that curves less than 30° at skeletal maturity tend to be stable through life, while curves over 40° are increasingly unstable and more likely to drift over time. This is largely caused by gravity affecting structural changes in vertebrae and soft tissue. Several research studies support the use of scoliosis-specific physical therapy exercises (and sometimes braces) for the adult population as a method for pain management. We have younger and older adults with large magnitude, high risk curves who choose to wear a custom brace as part of their scoliosis management strategy.

It's important to note that certain curve patterns where the head is not aligned over the pelvis are more likely to progress over time causing pain and degeneration. In our experience, short term bracing interventions for decompensated curves should be considered for younger, skeletally mature teens and adults (16-22 years old) even if Cobb angle values are small. Although not widely understood or accepted, this protocol specifically focuses to retrain the vestibular function and improve proper spinal alignment and overall balance.

Grant Wood MS, CPO (UK), CO (US)

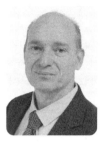

Grant Wood *specializes in three-dimensional bracing. He has the unique qualification of having trained and mentored with Dr. Manuel Rigo and Dr. Jacque Chêneau since 1995. Through the years, he has collaborated with them on numerous research publications, studies and workshops on the Chêneau Brace with the advanced Rigo principles. Grant Wood's professional career as an orthotist and prosthetist spans work in England, Spain, and his current US west coast practice in San Mateo, CA (align-clinic.com).*

What is a three-dimensional brace?

A three-dimensional brace refers to the shape. When looking down into the brace you will see there are large expansion areas. The brace is designed with built-in pressure and expansion areas to provide correction in all three planes of the body—coronal, sagittal and axial. Without these expansion areas/rooms, one cannot achieve optimal 3D correction, an important component, as this specific brace reinforces the correction that people learn while doing the Schroth Method exercises.

What's important to look for in an orthotist who is making a three-dimensional Rigo Chêneau–type brace?

First and foremost, it should be their reputation followed by individual skills, knowledge and experience. Any orthotist, no matter how good or certified they may be, will need years of experience to learn how to make a proper brace. This is especially true for an orthotist who makes a Rigo brace (three-dimensional) which depends even more heavily on an orthotist's familiarity with its principles to obtain favorable results. A scoliosis brace is not just an orthopedic product, but a device that is custom-made. It has to be highly specific to correct in 3D the trunk and spinal deformities, just as the old masters had done. Therefore, if the orthotist hasn't been personally hand-making, fabricating and fitting the Rigo Chêneau brace for at least five-to-seven years, on a regular basis, then I would question their ability to problem-solve many situations that will occur. And lastly, remember the name of the brace doesn't necessarily make it a good brace.

What is your approach when you brace a patient?

The goal is to create a brace shape that truly acknowledges all the dimensions of the patient's body, not just for today, but for the rest of their life. As an orthotist, this means not to be short-sighted and fixated on one number. This may require forfeiting a larger in-brace correction in order to have a better out-of-brace result —clinically and radiologically.

How does three-dimensional bracing differ in design from the standard TLSO?

The standard TLSO brace is more or less a full-contact and symmetrical brace, while the three-dimensional brace is not. The Chêneau Rigo-modified brace views scoliosis as a three-dimensional condition, addressing all three planes, not just one. I have seen many cases in which professionals have pushed the thoracic curve so much (sandwich effect) that it was disadvantageous to the two other planes. Therefore, the concepts I use might accept less Cobb correction while improving corrections in the other planes and other curves. The Cobb angle is important to me, but I am not going to negatively affect other planes (increase the flatback and rotation) and provide a poor clinical presentation at the cost of improved Cobb angle.

Do you just work with the three-dimensional brace?

No. As an orthotist, I have been trained to fit and fabricate all manner of braces for various scoliosis conditions—infantile, upper thoracic curves, neuromuscular, as well as for adults with scoliosis.

My master's thesis specialization is with the Rigo-modified Chêneau TLSO for scoliosis. I treat patients who have been prescribed Boston, Providence, Charleston, and other types of TLSO braces. However, with Dr. Rigo as my mentor, I made Rigo-modified Chêneau braces in Spain for eight years. This is the type of brace that most of my patients have and it is my preferred brace for most curves. This is not to say that other TLSOs if well-fitted and well-constructed are not efficacious. The Chêneau Rigo-modified braces, including the Wood Chêneau Rigo, is my choice because it addresses the three-dimensional nature of the curve, rather than just correcting the Cobb angle.

WCR brace designs have been presented in many different case presentations at: align-clinic.com/casepresentations-437506.html

What would you consider a good in-brace correction?

That depends on the individual clinical presentation. For example, if a patient is more skeletally mature and presents with larger curves, it would be unrealistic to expect a 50% in-brace correction. It could happen but no one can promise this. In-brace Cobb angle correction should not be the sole determining factor of how successful a brace is or is not because it only measures one aspect of the scoliosis curve. Too much focus on the in-brace Cobb angle result can lead to applying forces in a way that might improve the Cobb angle correction but negatively affect the scoliosis as a whole. This problem has occurred with non-bracing traction techniques as well.

Is physical therapy recommended in conjunction with this brace?

Yes. The Schroth-based Rigo Method taught by Dr. Manuel Rigo at the Barcelona Scoliosis Physiotherapy School (BSPTS) as well as International Schroth Scoliosis Therapy (ISST), are highly recommended as an adjunct to the Chêneau Rigo-modified brace. Many people now claim to treat scoliosis with Schroth therapy. I ask my patients to make sure they are seeing someone who was trained and certified by the BSPTS or ISST. These therapies have incorporated breathing exercises and postural corrections into the curriculum that work hand-in-glove with these types of braces. Schroth-certified PTs can modify any exercise for a different TLSO, but the exercises were created and have evolved with the Chêneau Rigo-modified brace.

How does the WCR brace address high thoracic curves?

Over the last several years, we have created an additional 3-point pressure brace that can treat very high curves or proximal structural thoracic curves. The brace design depends on the level of the upper thoracic curve apex.

For an apex of T3-4, we use a superstructure which is a thin piece of plastic that goes over the patient's shoulder to produce a downward pressure on the convex upper thoracic side, which controls the curve progression. This is a removable piece that is to be worn approximately 1 hour per day while sitting upright.

We can treat curves at the T5 level, as well as address curves higher by adding a "D modifier" incorporated into the shape of the brace. This allows re-inclination of the patient's shoulder on the convex thoracic side of the curve. The re-inclination is referring to having the shoulder move back and slightly down. Therefore, the shape of the brace and the direction of forces to the spine are different when compared with a standard WCR brace (a brace without the D-mod). The idea is to allow correction of the scoliosis without pushing on the spine in a way that would increase the upper thoracic curve.

Can you describe a couple of challenging corrections you were able to achieve?
There have been many great corrections the WCR brace has been able to obtain. One correction was a Cobb degree of 30° that achieved an in-brace correction of 2°, with an out-of-brace correction of 8°.

Another correction involved a four-year-old boy diagnosed with infantile scoliosis. His curve was 76° when his mother first contacted me following a failed brace treatment. I was able to obtain an out-of-brace correction of 45°, along with a significant improvement in the clinical appearance of the child's spine. Nine years later the child continues to do well. At 13 years old, his scoliosis is stable. His curves are now 35° out-of-brace, down from 76° pre-WCR brace and presents clinically very well. He has a much-improved scoliosis and quality of life and thus far has been able to avoid surgery.

Please note that this result is not always expected and does not necessarily mean that he won't require surgery in the future.

Can a scoliosis curve be treated with a nighttime brace exclusively?
In my opinion this is one of the biggest misunderstandings in bracing. It is the belief that a scoliosis that has a high risk of progression can be treated as effectively with a nighttime-only brace. The risk of progression dictates the wearing schedule of the patient, not the name of the brace. Therefore, we should not treat a high-risk scoliosis with a nighttime-only brace.

Do all braces help derotate the curve?
This is a complicated question because I don't think many orthotists would say that the brace they make or provide doesn't derotate. In fact, a symmetrical Boston-type brace might derotate. If you put an asymmetrical body into a symmetrical brace, it would derotate some by a "sandwich" effect, from squeezing the body together. However, in those

types of braces, the derotation will quickly rotate back after the brace has been removed.

To truly derotate a complex scoliosis, we must have a carefully designed brace with the forces at the correct levels and locations, and the correct amount of push pressure from the brace. The expansion areas are actual significant spaces (not "windows") in the brace. This is where most braces cut corners and fall short of a true 3D correction and true asymmetrical brace characteristics.

I presented a clear and simple explanation of this during the SOSORT 2019 San Francisco preconference meeting, which is available to watch on SOSORT.org under the videos section.

Is wearing a brace for patients with larger curves, such as 45°–55°, more uncomfortable?

No. If the brace is designed and modified correctly, it should be comfortable. Often I have patients who after wearing the brace for a couple weeks feel that it is more comfortable wearing the brace. However, if it is designed and fit incorrectly, then it would be more uncomfortable for any curve.

Can a 3D brace be helpful for a skeletally mature young adult with scoliosis?

Yes. The adult WCR brace is used for adults with moderate to severe scoliosis. It is designed to reduce pain, provide alignment of the pelvis and trunk, and improve aesthetics and postural control. The improved alignment of the pelvis and trunk reduces the imbalance of forces to the spine, which helps to control or slow the progression of the scoliosis.

When the WCR adult scoliosis brace is chosen, it is essential to assemble an experienced team of scoliosis professionals that include an orthopedic surgeon, a physical therapist trained in the Rigo Method, and an orthotist.

James Wynne CPO, FAAOP

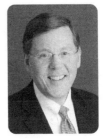

Jim Wynne is Vice President - Director of Education/Resident Director for Boston Orthotics and Prosthetics (bostonoandp. com). Jim has been a certified orthotist/prosthetist since 1991 and has specialized in pediatric orthotic/prosthetics, since 1993. He lectures both nationally and internationally on the non-operative management of scoliosis and has authored several book chapters and peer review articles on the non-operative treatment of scoliosis. He is the past president of the American Board for Certification in Orthotics, Prosthetics and Pedorthics and served as President for the Society on Scoliosis Orthopedic and Rehabilitation Treatment (SOSORT), the International Society on Scoliosis Orthopedic and Rehabilitation Treatment.

What is important for a parent to know about Boston Orthotics & Prosthetics (Boston O & P) braces?

The Boston brace was created in the 1970s by our founder, Bill Miller, along with top orthopedic specialists as a new way of treating scoliosis.

It's important for parents to know that Boston O & P is clinic-based. That is how our company started—with an orthotist being part of the clinical team, treating patients. All the innovations came from working with both our own clinicians, as well as those seeing patients in other clinics. Our approach has evolved with our improved knowledge of scoliosis along with the advent of new scanning and a computer software system that allows us to design the most appropriate and biomechanically sound brace. Each brace is custom-made, from individually carved models of the patient. We constantly look at how our patients are doing to ensure they achieve the best result and to learn how to improve each day. Boston O & P is all about helping kids one at a time.

After 50 years, it has been the most studied scoliosis brace and remains one of the leading non-operative braces for treating scoliosis.

From your experience, how important is the orthotist-patient relationship?

Very important. We did a study asking previous wearers about their experience. Many stated how supportive the orthotist was and that they wanted to wear their brace because of how dedicated the person was in helping them through the process.

Generally, what amount of in-brace correction should a parent expect when their child has their first X-ray?

Typically, we see 50 – 70% in-brace correction for single curves and 40 – 50% for double curves. But these are averages, and there are many variables that determine what's possible with in-brace correction including but not limited to: the stage the patient is at, location of the curve(s), and flexibility of the curve(s). We also look at general curve types to give us some guidance on what we can expect. The literature tells us we should maximize the curve correction while maintaining the patient's overall balance (shoulders level, not leaning to one side or to the front or back)—all while ensuring the patient can wear the brace.

Do you prefer to take an in-brace X-ray the day the child receives their brace or wait several weeks for her body to adjust?

Our protocol is to wait a few weeks after the fitting to obtain the in-brace X-ray. We feel this allows the patient time to break into the brace and for the curve to "stretch out." Also, the patient's torso (because of the soft tissue) will conform a bit to the brace and the brace will close down during the first few weeks of wear. We like to see our patients before the first in-brace X-ray to see how the break-in wear schedule is going and to make adjustments to the brace. Sometimes we add/remove specific padding and/or trim areas for comfort.

Are there benefits of having straps in the front versus the back of the brace?

Biomechanical studies show there is no difference. We do both front and back opening. Our patients are able to put the brace on themselves regardless. Patients with the straps on the back say they like it because they don't want the straps showing in the front. Either way is fine.

Do you think a brace monitor, such as iButton, can increase brace compliance?

Yes. The iButton is an electronic device that records temperature. It is very low profile, about the size of a dime. It snaps into the brace and records the temperature at certain intervals.

A recent study showed that patients who knew their wear schedule was being monitored had better adherence to the recommended wear schedule than those that did not know they were monitored. Since dose (number of hours the brace is worn) is the key to success, anything that increases adherence is important to incorporate into the treatment.

Part 4: Understanding the World of Bracing

Our experience has been that patients will wear the brace if they are comfortable. If they reach the recommended wear time, great; if they are having some challenges, we talk about it with the objective data. We can see the average daily pattern, so we can discuss and develop individual strategies. It's all about teamwork. Our patients and parents have found this device and method to be useful, as well as effective in monitoring brace wear.

What is the cost for such a device and can it be installed in any brace?

We offer the iButton to our families at no charge. They can opt in or out—their choice. No judgement.

Yes, the iButton can be installed in any style of brace, at any time during the treatment phase. It just needs to be within 3–5mm of the body. The same iButton can be used on the patient's second brace, if needed. Since there is only so much data storage on the iButton, it needs to have the existing data downloaded periodically in order to continue to collect new data.

Most patients want to see their brace wear report and are proud of their hard work.

How do you evaluate effective bracing?

We can look at a lot of things and we want to make sure we are not just pointing to the patient. We know that the ability to wear the brace is paramount, so we need to make sure that the brace is as comfortable as possible while still being effective. The ideal brace provides for good sagittal balance, curve reduction, rotational improvement and does not impede respiration. We like having the ability to adjust our padding and areas of relief accordingly, in order to maintain these goals during the patient's bracing journey. This is evaluated during consistent follow-up visits as part of the program.

Have you seen successful outcomes when bracing 45°-50° curves?

The short answer is yes. We have many single patient case studies showing positive results. But, as stated above, it depends. Single long curves of this magnitude may respond. Scoliosis is not just the value of the curve but the twist (rotation) that creates a rib prominence. Curves of this magnitude may have a large rib prominence which bracing can help along with scoliosis-specific exercises, but it depends on the curve.

Unlike the long single curve of this magnitude, a relatively short curve (meaning not many vertebrae are involved) can be a challenge. Another factor for success depends on the amount of growth remaining with concern for the potential rate of progression in adulthood.

Tell us the difference, if any, in effectiveness between the original Boston Brace and Boston 3D?

There are many long-term studies showing the effectiveness of the original Boston Brace, meaning some patients wearing the original not only prevented their curve from progressing, but saw curve improvement in the initial years after bracing. Today, with the advancements in technology, we are able to use body scanners to capture the patient's shape. That shape is then uploaded into our computer program to be modified. This has replaced the need to cast the patient and hand modify.

The Boston Brace 3D is custom-made from a scan of the patient. We are seeing an improvement in the initial in-brace corrections, while allowing us to not compress the abdomen, and not change the patient's sagittal (side view) profile. You may see older photos of the Boston Brace where the belly is compressed and the patient is leaning forward. That is not true today. The Boston 3D is an enhancement of the Boston Brace Principles; we build in many of the forces and enhance the relief areas to allow the patient to shift into the voids more. The combination of scanning the patients and providing them objective data regarding their wear time has improved our results. Many patients doing scoliosis-specific exercises (Schroth and the like) find it easier to do their exercise with these enhanced voids.

Can Boston Brace 3D address higher thoracic curves?

Yes, but it again depends. For apexes above the shoulder blades, it's harder because we do not have much leverage. We change the shape and position of the highest part of the brace that sits under the patient's arm. We sometimes extend the back section or create a front piece off the underarm extension. Since all the braces are custom, we fabricate what is best for the patient.

Does Boston Orthotics & Prosthetics also fabricate a nighttime brace?

Yes, the Boston Night Shift is our nocturnal brace. It, too, is a custom-form scan. It does not bend the spine in the opposite direction; it brings the spine to neutral. We are seeing very positive results. Because it is custom-made, we support the sagittal plane in a lying down position. For patients that have mild curves, are weaning out of bracing, or have a difficult time in fulltime bracing, it is an option.

Can you elaborate on the effectiveness of scoliosis-specific exercises with the Boston 3D brace?

We presented a poster at the 2019 SOSORT Conference showcasing the effectiveness of a combined treatment approach: *Boston Brace 3D and Scoliosis - Specific Exercises.* This poster highlighted a 14-year-old female who was observed over the course of two years. Her Cobb angle began at 49° in November of 2017. After diligently wearing her Boston Brace 3D for 18 hours a day and practicing her scoliosis-specific exercises (20-30 minutes a day, five days a week), her Cobb angle was reduced to 11° by August 2019.

I am happy to say we have many other successful stories from this team approach.

As an added bonus, we were also awarded "top poster" by our peers at the end of the SOSORT International Conference—a recognition we were very honored and proud to have received.

PART 5

Physical Therapy Scoliosis Specific Exercises

By now, you've probably talked to medical professionals about your daughter's care and likely heard that she should be braced for some period of time—and that if the brace doesn't produce measurable results, surgery should be considered.

For more than 100 years, the standard of care for scoliosis in the United States has been observation, bracing and surgery. But in other parts of the world, the emphasis has been on conservative care options such as Physical Therapy (Physiotherapy) Scoliosis Specific Exercises (PSSE).

While working on the first edition of Straight Talk with the Curvy Girls, PSSE was not well known in the US, with few practitioners available. But times are changing and these conservative treatments are increasingly making their way into the main-stream. Awareness continues to grow, and so, too, are the number of physical therapists certified to provide this care. For the purpose of this section, we will explore three types of scoliosis-specific exercises that are currently practiced in the US.

We hope you take the time to learn about these viable and non-invasive treatment options.

Rigo Method

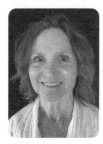

Beth Janssen, PT, co-founder of Scoliosis Rehab (scoliosisrehab.com), the first physical therapy clinic in the US dedicated to the treatment of scoliosis, in Stevens Point, Wi. Beth has been a practicing physical therapist since 1986, when she graduated from the Mayo School of Health-Related Sciences in Rochester, MN. She has worked extensively in hospital settings, where her practice focused on evaluation and treatment of spinal and TMJ dysfunction, women's health problems, scoliosis rehabilitation, and mentoring of new physical therapists. She has done advanced studies in the McKenzie approach to treating spinal dysfunction, along with Muscle Energy Techniques and Myofascial Release training. In 2003, she was trained in the conservative care of scoliosis with Dr. Manuel Rigo. In 2015, she expanded her clinic to San Jose, Ca. Today, Beth continues her working relationship with Dr. Rigo and the methods that are now referred to as BSPTS – Rigo Method.

How did you learn there was scoliosis-specific exercises for scoliosis?

When my son was diagnosed with scoliosis, I didn't think I could passively "watch and wait" to see if his condition deteriorated. So I began researching other treatments for scoliosis. I learned about the Schroth Method when I read Martha Hawes' book, *Scoliosis and the Human Spine*. In this book, she mentions an exercise model, the Schroth Method, which has been used successfully in Germany for over one hundred years. After reading her book, I called Germany to see if I could attend the Asklepios Schroth clinic with my son. They sent me to Dr. Rigo in Spain, where the patients were taught in English. While my son was receiving treatment from Dr. Rigo, I also became trained and certified in the Schroth Method.

Having seen the benefits of Schroth therapy, I was passionate about utilizing the techniques in the job I held at a local hospital. But in the hospital setting, most physical therapy departments don't specialize in a single type of patient. I began to think that other physical therapists in the US needed to learn about Schroth if they had the opportunity to work with a person with scoliosis.

At my request, in 2005, Dr. Rigo did the first training course in the US for physical therapists in Stevens Point, Wisconsin. I was the clinical assistant for this ten-day course, which certified several other physical therapists here. In 2006, we opened Scoliosis Rehab Inc, so I could concentrate on this patient population.

In* Straight Talk Scoliosis *first edition you spoke about your PT practice using the Schroth Method. Is that what you are practicing today?

I think to answer this question we need to look historically at the evolution of PSSE. I was certified in the Schroth Method in 2003 by Dr Rigo, who had taught Schroth since the 1980's. As time went on, he clarified techniques and added principles that are more clearly defined. These changes reflect his personal experiences as a physician, clinician and teacher. In 2009, when he left the Schroth teaching group, he began to teach his evolved method. What I practice today is the BSPTS-Rigo Method, which has evolved from Schroth.

Can you explain the concept of the Rigo Method?

The Rigo Method is one of the seven Physiotherapy Scoliosis Specific Exercise (PSSE) schools known around the world with scientific proof of effectiveness in treating scoliosis. Based on the original work by Katharina Schroth, the Rigo Method promotes stability of the corrective posture. This concept is part of a comprehensive treatment program that involves a team approach including, the patient and family member, physician trained in the treatment of spinal disorders, physical therapist (PT), orthotist, and counselor, as needed.

How is the Rigo Method taught?

This method uses specific postural corrections based on an individual's curve pattern based on sensorimotor and kinesthetic principles. That means patients have to develop a self-awareness of where their bodies are in space, how they hold their bodies now, and how they should actually be holding their bodies.

The patient learns the corrected posture by actually practicing moving the body through space and holding this reformed position. The PT works with the patient to help develop this self-awareness in three dimensions. The Rigo Method trains the person to correct the scoliotic posture with proprioceptive and external stimulation and mirrors.

Proprioceptive stimulation means that you have to perceive where your body is in space, relative to the other parts of your body, and be aware of the effort needed to move the body into the more balanced alignment. The external stimulation is initially the hands of a well-trained PT guiding the treatment, and also the pads and props used by the therapist. Eventually, as deeper self-awareness is developed, the patient can find the corrected position independently and maintain it at least partially in daily life.

The patients use an individually developed routine of corrections to lift themselves out of the curve pattern in three dimensions, along with a new breathing pattern to further expand concave or collapsed areas. With these new positions, we are correcting as much of the postural collapse as possible, in order to decrease the mechanical forces that may be contributing to the progression of the curve.

What Cobb degree can treatment begin?

We follow the SOSORT guidelines. In order to not over-treat, we usually begin this program at a 15° Cobb angle, based on the chance of progression. If there is any pain or other problems present, we may begin at a smaller Cobb angle. Also, if there is a strong family history of scoliosis, we may recommend bracing or physical therapy intervention earlier than we would when there is no history.

Is there an age requirement?

We follow the BSPTS guidelines. This recommendation includes waiting until the child is ten years old for girls and twelve years old for boys. Since girls enter their pubertal growth spurt before boys, we want to give them the information that they need when they are actively growing. Committing to this program requires a certain level of developmental maturity in order to be able to focus on posture and alignment. Also, if we start too young, we risk having them burn out before they hit the most critical time of growth (puberty), when the curve is more likely to progress.

What should a new patient expect during their initial visit?

On the first visit, the physical therapist reviews the patient's medical history and does a comprehensive evaluation with a postural assessment. Upon reviewing the radiologic information, the clinical findings are then clarified. The curve pattern will then be categorized using the Rigo Classification. Individual characteristics of the curve, along with other orthopedic needs of the patient will be addressed.

A treatment plan will be proposed to the patient and family, which will take into consideration the dynamic family needs, including psychological and social aspects. The plan will be discussed and continuously modified until it is agreed upon.

Once treatment begins, a plan is then sent to the physician so a team approach can be facilitated. Contact will be made with the orthotist if needed. The specific physical therapy treatment plan proposed by the evaluating PT is based on the findings of the evaluation. Studies have shown that when the team approach is used, patient compliance is improved.[1]

The therapist then proceeds to educate the patient and family on anatomy, the three-dimensional nature of scoliosis and the individual posture, body mechanics, and the vicious cycle[2] that could worsen their posture if left unchecked.

What should a patient expect during follow-up visits?

After the patient has a sense of how the spine curves and how that affects their posture, the PT moves onto teaching specific new positions. We follow these principles: perform 3D postural correction with movement, then expand with breath support, stabilize in their new corrective posture, and finally learn to integrate the new posture into their daily life.

This is a very interactive process in which the patient learns the corrected posture position while the PT watches the exercise and modifies, as needed. Once this is well understood and performed independently, the patient will then be taught additional positions based on their own abilities and needs. The program is a tool to learn the new posture.

When can a person begin to see a change?

As far as a person noticing a change, this varies depending on the individual. Most people with myofascial pain will feel a positive change within a short period of time. If there are some secondary problems, such as arthritic changes, or disc issues combined with pressure on the nerves, the exercises may or may not help the pain.

---

[1] Stefano Negrini (2008) "Approach to scoliosis changed due to causes other than evidence: Patients call for conservative (rehabilitation) experts to join in team orthopedic surgeons." *Disability and Rehabilitation*, 30:10, 731-741, DOI: 10.1080/09638280801889485

[2] Stokes, I.A., Burwell, R.G. & Dangerfield, P.H. "Biomechanical spinal growth modulation and progressive adolescent scoliosis – a test of the 'vicious cycle' pathogenetic hypothesis: Summary of an electronic focus group debate of the IBSE." *Scoli*osis 1, 16 (2006). (scoliosisjournal.biomedcentral.com)

Most adolescents' receiving intensive training will see changes in the shape of their torso within the first week. This positive change will happen when the patient does the muscle activation. Once a person sinks back into their old posture, the change will be gone. The longer the patient remains in the corrected posture, the easier it becomes to find the corrected posture and stay there.

By using these concepts, the PT is trying to teach patients a new way to hold themselves in three dimensions. We work to have the patient recognize what the corrected position feels like and then to know how to stabilize the body in this new position.

What are realistic long-term changes a patient can expect?

The long-term changes that can be achieved will be dependent on the individual situation of each patient. Realistic goals should be discussed and agreed upon at the time of the evaluation while considering all of the evidence, along with the skill of the physical therapist and the desires of the patient and family. For example, a 17-year-old girl with AIS and a 48° Cobb angle with the expectation of achieving a straight spine would not be realistic. But if that patient and family have a goal of learning how to care for her back, stabilize her curve, improve her posture, and control any pain—in many cases, that could be achievable.

During our program we also teach posture and body mechanics with a neutral spine. We also develop a scoliosis-specific home exercise program based upon the curve pattern, as well as individual characteristics of the patient and their biopsychosocial needs.

What does it mean to keep your spine in neutral?

Spinal neutral means holding the back in a position where from the side view you have the normal curves of the back, lordosis (a curve going inward) at the neck and low back, and kyphosis (a curve going backward) at the rib cage. It also means that the pelvis is balanced in a left-to-right position, leveled and not rotated. This is something that we teach in therapy and sometimes it takes extensive training to learn.

A person should try to keep the back more or less straight with a small inward curve in the low back without twisting or side bending. This neutral posture should be the goal during most daily activities. Because many people with scoliosis do not feel like they are standing in an uneven posture, learning to stand and sit in neutral may require repetition. Moving with a neutral spine is a principle that is used to help many people with spinal problems besides scoliosis. Keeping the spine in neutral promotes disc health by keeping the pressure on the discs more balanced.

Does Rigo Method require full-time bracing?

We advocate part-time or full-time bracing for adolescents based on the magnitude of the Cobb angle, skeletal maturity, and risk of progression from other known factors, such as family history. The decision to brace is made on a case-by-case basis, ideally by a multidisciplinary team and following SOSORT guidelines. If bracing is indicated, PSSE alone is not enough to stabilize the curve.

If you are braced and perform these exercises, can curves still progress?

These individually crafted scoliosis-specific physical therapy regimens when performed in conjunction with bracing have, in some cases, been an effective treatment to halt or stabilize idiopathic adolescent scoliosis and, in some cases, reverse the scoliosis curvature. However, in some cases, no matter if the child has the best brace and PT program, the curve may progress.

Is the Rigo Method taught one-on-one or in a group?

As per SOSORT recommendations, PSSE should be taught individually because each patient's spinal curve, rotation, degree of trunk imbalance, muscle condition, and patient need is unique. In this way, we are able to tailor the physical therapy program to each patient's specific needs.

At Scoliosis Rehab, when a patient comes for an intensive one- to two-week session, we offer them some time to practice their therapy in what we refer to as "Open Gym." During Open Gym, the patients work independently at the skill level that they have achieved and report back to the PT at the next session. In this way we can address areas of confusion or concern. It is also possible once the patient is well trained that they can join a small group of trained patients, under the supervision of the PT to work together on a maintenance program.

Can PSSE benefit patients that have been fused?

It is important for a surgically-fused individual to understand where their bodies are in space: Is the pelvis balanced or out to one side? Are the shoulders balanced over the rib cage? Are the shoulders level? Is the head tilted or forward? Is the breathing pattern altered?

The program can be modified for the patients who have had surgery. This is for those who may need to improve symmetry, balance, flexibility, core stabilization and address pain. These concepts are taught through postural alignment and to assist with a more specific breathing pattern.

After surgery, all of the movement that would have been distributed throughout the spine now only occurs above and below the fusion, so it is essential to consider the "wear and tear" at the ends of the fused site. We encourage low-impact activities with the spine in neutral to prolong the health of the post-surgical back. In some ways, it is even more important for a person with a fusion to understand how to take care of their back.

Are there any exercises that are not healthy for a scoliotic spine?

Yes. Exercises that move the spine out of neutral could be detrimental, but this is dependent on the severity of the curve. This should be discussed individually with your PT. We generally advocate for people with scoliosis to do their exercises with the spine in neutral.

With idiopathic scoliosis, the vertebral bodies of the main curve become wedge-shaped—some vertebrae are taller in the front than the back, and taller on the convex (rib or lumbar prominence) side of the curve than on the concave side. There is also usually some collapse in the concave areas.

When people with idiopathic scoliosis bend forward, the prominences become more noticeable. This flexion causes increased torsion in the spine, which then pushes the spine more into the pattern of the scoliosis. The wedge shape of the thoracic vertebrae can lead to loss of thoracic kyphosis, which is a loss of the normal shape of the spine when viewed from the side. In some people with scoliosis, the thoracic spine can actually become flat or go into lordosis (an inward curve of the spine when looking at the side view). So when a person with scoliosis does backward bending (or extension), they push the spine forward, which exaggerates the forward push on the thoracic spine causing a reduction in thoracic kyphosis. We want a certain amount of kyphosis in the thoracic spine because it provides stability and allows room for the heart and lungs.

Just as flexion increases the torsion of the spine, and extension decreases the stability of the spine, side bending can increase the size of the lateral curve(s). In scoliosis, one curve doesn't generally exist alone; most often there is at least a small compensatory curve above or below the primary curve. We teach that daily movements and exercises are to be performed with the spine in neutral in 3D with self-elongation.

> We do not advocate side bending or rotational exercises because when you move into side bending or rotation, you will be straightening one curve but feeding into the other curve.

Is there an impact on curves when doing push-ups and crunches?

Push-ups are fine as long as the person can keep their trunk in neutral. We advocate that all exercises be done with the spine in neutral as described above. We have other abdominal exercises that we teach instead of crunches. These exercises can strengthen the abdominals without increasing the torsion of the spine or feeding into the pattern of the scoliosis.

What about participation in exercise programs such as yoga and Pilates?

Yoga and Pilates have some valuable elements. They are calming, promote deep breathing and require attention to alignment. But for either of these disciplines, we suggest that the spine is held in neutral and if you are trained in PSSE, we suggest that you do your 3D postural correction first, and then do the Pilates or yoga while maintaining that corrected alignment.

If someone wants to participate in community-based exercises they should seek to understand their scoliosis through PSSE prior to the class. I would also recommend that they follow the advice of a PT certified in PSSE as defined by SOSORT.

What is the difference between working with a BSPTS physical therapist versus yoga or Pilate's instructor?

The formal training of a physical therapist is much more extensive than an instructor for yoga or Pilate's. It is based on a unique body of knowledge supported by educational preparation on research and clinical evidence (pta.org). Entry level education for PTs is now a doctoral degree. Also, all physical therapists require a state licensure in order to practice, but it is not a universal prerequisite for yoga or Pilates instructors.

The scope of practice of physical therapists includes examining X-rays to determine if certain radiology findings are present, which make an exercise appropriate or harmful. Reviewing radiological findings is not in the scope of practice for a yoga or Pilate's instructor.

What exercises can you recommend for general fitness?

First of all, we should all select general fitness exercises that bring us joy. If you love to run and you can't be happy without it, then run, but only run with good form and do it in moderation. If stopping soccer is going to make you sad—play soccer, but invest in your health and do exercises specifically to care for your spine. We all need aerobic training and perhaps low impact aerobic exercises. Walking, biking, swimming and elliptical training are the best.

Most importantly, awareness of how you move your spine when performing any exercise is essential. For most people with scoliosis, when your body becomes fatigued, the natural tendency is to slump back into the scoliotic posture. The patient should exercise when they feel they can maintain proper posture.

Why do some curves progress after skeletal maturity?

The most probable cause of curve progression after a person is skeletally mature is that they are used to the posture of the scoliosis. The body is fixed in the uneven position from the structural scoliosis. If they don't have a strategy to move themselves out of the curve in three dimensions, then they stay there. The tight tissues stay tight and those tissues that have lengthened out to accommodate the curvature remain lengthened. This is supported by the Vicious Cycle model proposed by Stokes.[3]

The mechanical forces, originating from the uneven load on the trunk from the curve, interacting with gravity and movements of daily life, slowly push the person more into the curve. This can happen slowly a little each day, week, or year, causing the spine to slowly collapse into the curve. This is more likely to happen in curves that exceed a certain Cobb angle.

What long-term goals do you want patients to achieve?

A patient with scoliosis often finds it most comfortable to stand in a posture that reinforces the scoliosis curvatures. The objective is to learn the

---

[3] Stokes, I.A., Burwell, R.G. & Dangerfield, P.H. Biomechanical spinal growth modulation and progressive adolescent scoliosis – a test of the 'vicious cycle' pathogenetic hypothesis: Summary of an electronic focus group debate of the IBSE. *Scoli*osis 1, 16 (2006). (scoliosisjournal.biomedcentral.com)

new corrected position so completely that they automatically maintain this corrected posture to some degree as they go through activities of daily life.

The goal for a patient trained in this method is to stand in a non-scoliotic posture and, with practice, to be able to subconsciously assume the corrected posture rather than the collapsed scoliotic posture throughout their life. We believe that will result in back health that is permanently better for the patient.

Who is qualified to provide PSSE?

According to SOSORT guidelines, a physical therapist specifically trained in PSSE is qualified. These are physical therapy programs for scoliosis that have significant research to support their effectiveness as defined by SOSORT.

The prospective patient or a family member should ask the clinician when the physical therapist was certified. It is important to ensure they actively practice this method by asking how many scoliosis patients this therapist treats annually.

What is involved in becoming certified?

The training in the method has recently been modified to ensure a good mix of theory and practical hands-on training. The website BSPTS. net will describe the training required for physical therapists interested in the method. It includes 21 days of training spread over 1-3 years. There are requirements for the passing of written and practical examinations, observation hours and the presentation of a case report.

How do we find certified therapists in our area?

You can visit BSPTS.net for a list of trained physical therapists.

Does your clinic accept insurance?

Our clinic in Wisconsin does accept some types of insurance. Since first learning of this method in 2003, it has been a dream of mine to make this treatment accessible to people all over the country. We have made progress. Our teaching group has trained over 200 physical therapists since 2010. As a result, people no longer have to travel only to Europe for this treatment. With so many clinicians trained, you will find many different opportunities for insurance coverage or discounts for payment at the time of service. Thanks to our extensive training program, we now have certified physical therapists in many states, working in many clinics.

Are there any randomized controlled clinical trials supporting PSSE?

The following is a list of high-level studies that present the effectiveness of Physiotherapy Scoliosis Specific Exercise programs:

1. Zapata KA, Sucato DJ, Jo CH. (2019) "Physical Therapy Scoliosis-Specific Exercises May Reduce Curve Progression in Mild Adolescent Idiopathic Scoliosis Curves." *Pediatr Phys Ther*, Jul 31(3):280-285..

2. Schreiber S, Parent EC, Khodayari Moez E, Hedden DM, Hill DL, Moreau M, et al. (2016) "Schroth Physiotherapeutic Scoliosis-Specific Exercises Added to the Standard of Care Lead to Better Cobb Angle Outcomes in Adolescents with Idiopathic Scoliosis – An Assessor and Statistician Blinded Randomized Controlled Trial." *PLoS ONE*, 11(12): e0168746.

3. Kuru T, Yeldan İ, Dereli EE, Özdinçler AR, Dikici F, Çolak İ. (2016) "The efficacy of three-dimensional Schroth exercises in adolescent idiopathic scoliosis: a randomized controlled clinical trial." *Clin Rehabil*, Feb 30(2):181–90.

4. Kwan KYH, Cheng ACS, Koh HY, Chiu AYY, Cheung KMC. (2017) "Effectiveness of Schroth exercises during bracing in adolescent idiopathic scoliosis: results from a preliminary study: SOSORT Award 2017 Winner." *Scoliosis and Spinal Disorders*, Oct 16, 12:32.

Other supportive studies and information:

1. Marti C, et al. (2015) "Scoliosis Research Society members' attitudes towards physical therapy and physiotherapeutic scoliosis specific exercises for adolescent idiopathic scoliosis." *Scoliosis and Spine Disorders, 10(16)*.

2. Negrini A, Negrini MG, Donzelli S, Romano M, Zaina F, Negrini S. (2015) "Scoliosis- Specific exercises can reduce the progression of severe curves in adult idiopathic scoliosis: a long-term cohort study." *Scoliosis*, Jul 11, 10:20.

What are the currently accepted PSSE schools?

The current list of evidence-based schools includes BSPTS-Rigo Method (Barcelona), FITS and DOBOMED (Poland), SEAS (Italy), Schroth (Germany), Sideshift (England), Lyon (France), and Global Postural Reeducation (Canada).

All PSSE programs consist of auto-correction in 3D, training in activities of daily living, stabilizing the corrected posture, and patient education.

For a more in-depth description of the various PSSE schools, consider reading *Physiotherapy Scoliosis Specific Exercises* by H. Berdishevsky.

PERSONAL MESSAGE OF GRATITUDE:

I have been honored to meet and work with quite a few Curvy Girls. Many have embraced the method. Since 2010, when the first Curvy Girl was treated, most orthopedic surgeons were not familiar with this type of conservative treatment. Through CG advocacy this method has gained wide spread recognition across the country, among families and medical professionals.

—Beth Janssen

Setting It Straight

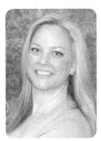

Marissa Muccio, PT, C/NDT, leads the largest clinic for Schroth in the US, Scoliosis Specialty Center (scoliosisspecialtycenter.com) in Mount Pleasant, SC. She graduated from the University of Medicine and Dentistry of New Jersey (Rutgers School of Biomedical and Health Sciences) in 1998 with a Bachelor's in Physical Therapy. She has worked in a variety of pediatric settings including NICU, neuromuscular, cranial facial, pediatric oncology, pediatric in-patient, outpatient, Aquatics, EIP and Schroth PSSE. In 2011, she became one of the first C2 certified therapists in the US for the 3D treatment of scoliosis via the Barcelona Scoliosis Physiotherapy School and is committed to expanding the research for scoliosis-specific exercises. Marissa is also the medical advisor for the nonprofit Curvy Girls Foundation.

Scoliosis is a condition that does not discriminate. Children who are diagnosed with scoliosis might also have academic learning disabilities, autism and neuromuscular diseases.

How would a Schroth physical therapist teach a child with special needs these complex exercises?

First, it is critical to have an open discussion with all parties: parents, child if possible, therapist, and physician. To be absolutely clear there is little to no research on the outcomes of Schroth treatment within neuromuscular scoliosis or with children with learning disabilities or other neurological concurring diagnoses. There are case studies at best. I would not anticipate any significant research in these areas. Neurology is a challenging area to structure research as patients can have such a wide range of variations and unique presentations of the same labeled condition.

As leaders in this area of application, here is our philosophy and clinical approach.

Schroth is a motor training program. If a physical therapist is well trained and practiced in Schroth AND has training within these additional diagnoses, there may be room for modifying the program and training the patient and parents on components of Schroth.

If strategies using verbal, manual, toys, parental, and/or PT can produce the muscle contractions that are appropriate for that Schroth pattern, then with practice, there may be room for corrective changes.

What about younger children?

Research is very limited on Schroth and juvenile or early onset scoliosis. Clinically, we have been modifying Schroth for children as young as three. Remember, the theory behind Schroth is training of an individual's motor skills. How we teach movement to children younger than 10 is already understood within motor learning research and pediatric physical therapy. If the same strategies described above can produce the muscle contractions that are appropriate for that Schroth pattern, then with practice, there may be room for corrective changes. Even within the original Schroth clinic in Germany there were young children following the Polio outbreak who received treatment for their scoliosis. I believe a five-year-old was actually on the original textbook cover.

SETTING THE RECORD STRAIGHT: True or False

Families often read a lot about scoliosis online. Below are the most commonly asked and misinformed topics regarding scoliosis.

If one leg is longer than the other, a child can develop scoliosis.

False. While it's true that AIS is a disease/condition of the spine, and very significant leg length differences may cause a functional shift in body/spine, it doesn't trigger the disease process. Leg length is determined through X-rays of the long bones and measurements. Common treatment if actually diagnosed with a difference can be adding a lift to the short side foot/shoe substituting for the height difference and should help equal out the floor biomechanics. A shoe lift is NOT appropriate for patients whose scoliosis has resulted in an asymmetrical alignment of the biomechanical chain from spine to pelvis to leg.

Within the AIS population, there are often postural and biomechanical changes to the lumbar spine/pelvis which can cause one side to "hike up" thus creating the appearance of a leg difference. In these cases, providing a lift would NOT be recommended. Of course, there may be a small number of patients that have both conditions.

Bad posture, or carrying heavy backpacks, cause scoliosis.

That's false, too. Again, this is a disease/condition. However, high frequency and intensity (weight) of postures and backpacks can impact compensatory movement patterns resulting from scoliosis change in the spinal position in space. It is not clear in research as to their impact on progression risk. Healthy posture and prudent use of backpacks are recommended for ALL children.

Scoliosis can only be developed if it is in the family.

False. Approximately 30% of adolescent idiopathic scoliosis patients have a family history of scoliosis. That means that 70% do not have a family history.

There are no limits to physical activity following recovery from spinal fusion surgery.

False. Although most patients return to full activities of daily living and sports, not ALL activities are possible following SOME types of surgeries. There are differences in fused levels. There may also be some limits in highly combative/contact sports. Each patient and family should have a clear discussion with their surgeon on any limits that may apply to their specific case/fusion.

Scoliosis does not cause back pain.

HUGE FALSE! In the majority of cases, scoliosis does not cause back pain. However, in approximately 30% of cases, it does! Now, we do not know if there are other undiagnosed conditions that may be occurring that causes pain. Also, there are compensation patterns that can develop in response to the structural shift in a spine with scoliosis that can cause biomechanical muscle pain.

The onset of a girl's menstruation means her major growth spurt is over.

Generally, true! A girl's peak velocity growth spurt typically occurs prior to menstruation—but it can continue past the onset of menstruation. This also does NOT mean that growth is complete; some skeletal growth can continue even after menstruation begins. And, there is continued risk of curve progression. Still, parents should know that the peak velocity growth for girls occurs prior to menstruation. Current research has shown that Sanders Test (hand X-ray) is more valid for bone age than any previous test.

The only way to accurately monitor curve progression is from the Risser – bone plate found in the pelvis.

False. Sanders hand X-ray has begun to provide more accurate skeletal maturity staging for peak velocity time period. Sander's ability to isolate the peak velocity stage is something that the Risser is not sensitive enough to do and as the Columbia University Orthopedics research has shown, the Risser may have more error than originally thought. We use Sanders whenever possible and advocate for it. Columbia's recent research has shown that the Risser has an approximate 40% error rate. Thus, the Sanders Test is best current measure for bone growth staging.

Once I have spinal fusion surgery, I no longer have scoliosis.

False. Once spine growth is complete, the disease progression is finished. But it will always be present. For those falling into the surgical range, fusion cannot completely return a spine to 0 or neutral. Some may get close. Also keep in mind that the variables that are within scoliosis will remain, such as low bone density, osteopenia, vitamin deficiencies, joint hypermobility, etc.

Introduction to SEAS

SEAS (Scientific Exercise Approach to Scoliosis) is an Italian-based, conservative exercise treatment based upon scientific research with scoliosis patients.

When asked about the founder, Professor Stefano Negrini, MD, of Milan, Italy explains, "In fact, ISICO (Italian Scientific Spine Institute) was started by my parents, Antonio Negrini and Nevia Verzini, who were both trainers, and my father was also a physiotherapist. I was just the scientist who was so lucky to be born into such a family and to have another clinical master and second professional father, physician Dr. Paolo Sibilla, who taught me the art of both bracing and scoliosis treatment."

Centro Scoliosis Negrini was the foundation for the development of exercises based upon a scientific approach for scoliosis and kyphosis treatment. As the years progressed, their approach improved as the Negrinis exchanged their information and experiences with the top scoliosis centers in six European countries, resulting in a collaborative effort in the study and research of scoliosis.

Professor Negrini continues the scientific work that his parents began. He and his colleagues study and evaluate new and innovative ways to improve the efficacy of SEAS to achieve optimum results for a scoliotic body.

Stefano Negrini MD
Milan, Italy

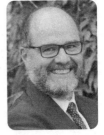

Dr. **Stefano Negrini** *is Scientific Medical Director and one of the founders of Italian Scientific Spine Institute (ISICO@isico.it), and SOSORT. He is full Professor in Physical and Rehabilitation Medicine at the University "La Statale" and Director of the Laboratory on Evidence-based Rehabilitation at the Orthopedic Institute Galezzi, Milan.*

Dr. Negrini is regarded as one of the most influential leaders in the rehabilitation of scoliosis and other spinal diseases. His vast research is primarily on evidence-based rehabilitation, with a focus on the efficacy of bracing and exercise for child and adolescent idiopathic scoliosis, and secondarily on conservative treatment of adult scoliosis, curve evaluation and classification, and lower back and neck pain. He has published over four hundred scientific papers, multiple abstracts, book chapters and textbooks on these topics. In addition, he was a founder of the Society on Scoliosis Orthopedic and Rehabilitation Treatment (SOSORT).

Can you explain what type of physician you are?

I'm a physician who specializes only in conservative (non-operative) treatment. In fact, I'm a physiatrist, which is a physical and rehabilitation medicine specialist, and not an orthopedic surgeon. Physical and Rehabilitation Medicine is the specialty which deals with the management of disabilities. In the area of spinal diseases, we often work on chronic lower back and neck pain, in combination with physical therapists. I strongly believe that we need specific expertise in either surgery or in conservative care. It's not possible today to stay at pace with progress in both of these areas. Orthopedic surgeons specializing in surgery presumably do not have the time to devote to the study of conservative treatment. The more surgical the orthopedic specialty has become, the more surgical were the options indicated for scoliosis patients by orthopedic surgeons.

How would you define conservative treatment?

Historically, conservative treatment has been defined by negation, meaning the application of all means other than surgery aimed at avoiding curve progression and potentially improving scoliosis. I prefer the term "rehabilitation treatment," but the term "conservative" is the standard and will remain as such until the various experts in this specialty come together to review the standard of care.

Today, we have evidence as to the efficacy of exercises and braces for scoliosis. We do not have evidence for manual therapy—chiropractic care, osteopathy, or traditional physical therapy modalities. Therefore, the term conservative treatment in the field of scoliosis refers only to exercises and bracing.

Can you describe SEAS?

SEAS principles are based on a specific form of auto-correction and active self-correction individualized to each patient's scoliosis, and then associated with stabilizing exercises including neuromotor control and proprioceptive training and balance.

Auto-correction is applied to all exercises aimed at reducing the functional impairment typical of scoliosis, and at minimizing the risk of progression.

Which movements are involved in SEAS auto-correction?

These exercises achieve derotation (trying to correct the vertebral rotation due to scoliosis), deflexion (reducing the scoliosis curve(s)), and restoration of the sagittal profile (fighting against the flat-back typical of the scoliosis and/or the kyphosis). A patient's specific scoliotic curve pattern and degrees will determine the exercises that are prescribed. Exercises are then adapted and tested for each patient.

What is the main goal of these exercises?

The goal of the exercises is training motor behavior, and developing self-awareness and reflex responses. This is what has been shown to be useful in our scoliosis patients. As much as possible, we use the active auto-correction. Other conservative methods may use physical aids throughout the course of treatment. SEAS only use aids at the beginning in order to speed up learning. Auto-correction is learned gradually over time. Like learning to dance, it takes practice. You cannot do it correctly immediately, and so we use some external aids during this learning phase.

How many patients do you treat per year?

I treat about one thousand patients conservatively per year. I meet each patient every four to six months for twenty to thirty minutes, and together with the orthotist for final brace checks.

During these visits, I not only evaluate, but also motivate patients to be compliant with their therapy and bracing. According to the SOSORT criteria, treating less than three hundred patients per year for brace treatment management, is not enough for specific expertise in this area.

At what curve degree do you begin SEAS?

On the average, we start at 15°. The first step is observation. Then, in an effort to avoid bracing, we start SEAS exercises as soon as we see significant risk factors for progression—such as curves greater than 15° or less than 15° with a significant hump or a flatback, a positive family history, or if the patient is in a rapid growth period. Conversely, if a person has reached physical maturity or has an insignificant hump with a curve higher than 15°, we can choose not to take any action. For us, decisions always come from many factors, not only Cobb degrees. If there are no other risk factors, we may not start at all. The process is fully personalized.

How often do you change a patient's exercise regime?

Exercises are modified on a regular basis every one to three months, according to the patient's growth, individual capacities, what has been learned, and so on. We adapt the exercises to what the patient is able to do and, consequently, the idea of "perfection" changes over time.

SEAS database consists of more than a thousand exercises which continue to be changed and adapted as we learn what is most effective. We also accept the idea that exercises will change completely according to new scientific discoveries. In this respect, SEAS is not a method but an approach. It is not closed nor fully codified. As we have changed in the past, we are sure to change again as new knowledge becomes available from both our own research, as well as from colleagues worldwide.

Do children who have successfully finished their bracing need to maintain an exercise program to prevent further curve progression?

No. Treatment must start and finish. Scoliosis patients need a healthy behavior like any other adult to maintain good physical fitness, which will definitely help their backs. If, however, the scoliosis progresses, we would need to restore specific exercises in order to try and avoid surgery.

What if the patient had a 45° curve at the end of treatment? Would the answer be the same?

No. If the scoliosis is above 45/50° and the patient did not want to consider surgery, exercises can help stabilize the curve. However, we would keep them under life-long observation in case we need to discuss other options in the future.

How do you address patients that experience treatment burnout?

We call this the "wash up" period, since most of the patients get tired of the long treatment and need to stop, if only for a little while. Observation continues, but prevention through exercises can wait. A few years of rest is not only psychologically healthier for these patients, but also allows for a change in mindset from therapy to prevention. We remind them that the time will come to once again focus on their scoliosis, knowing that adulthood will bring realization that exercises are beneficial for overall health, including scoliosis.

BRACING

In the US, the standard of care for bracing is when curves reach 25°. When do you begin bracing?

The decision to brace is determined by many factors, not only Cobb degree. We begin bracing with the soft braces (SpineCor®) between 20° and 30°. Rigid bracing begins between 25° to 30°.

In the US, bracing varies from 16 to 23 hours a day. How many hours do you recommend your patients brace per day?

Rigid braces can be prescribed 18 to 23 hours per day according to individual need. Our first aim is to reduce the burden on the patient, but this all depends on the scoliosis curve. The fewer hours, may be better for the patient, but riskier for curve progression.

The factors we consider in order to determine type of brace and wear hours include: Cobb degrees, period of growth (rapid or slow), bone age (young or mature), risk for progression (high versus low), type of curve, and physical structure of patient (thin or strong). When you use a more rigid brace, sometimes you can reduce the hours worn. However, this is not so simplistic since a spine that is curving aggressively needs to grow as much as possible in a correct position, which requires more hours of bracing per day.

How do you approach brace compliance in teens?

In my view, and that of SOSORT, obtaining compliance is mostly how the treating team approaches the patient. It is not just what you say to a patient but how you say it. We presented this in a SOSORT abstract in Barcelona, winning the SOSORT Award and published in Scoliosis Journal (scoliosisjournal.com), showing the highest compliance rates ever published—an average of almost 90%. This indicates that patients could be made to be compliant to bracing. If you want an asymptomatic teenager to wear plastic for years, you must believe in what you are doing, and you must apply all possible techniques to reinforce your message.

We also believe that the type of brace you wear plays a major role in terms of your overall success with bracing. Our braces are the most symmetrical in the literature, and we achieve results that are among the best published. We've been able to track compliance using sensors in the brace and found that adherence to prescribed treatment is more than 90%. We can't be sure about all the reasons for our high compliance rate. However, we do believe, that patients are more willing to wear our brace as prescribed because it's practically invisible to their peers.

What type of brace do you use?

We do not have one brace preference. In our clinics we have a variety of braces. Each brace is fully personalized and based on individual patient needs.

Our braces include a super-rigid Sforzesco brace for the most difficult situations, and a series of rigid: Sibilla brace (less rigid version of the Sforzesco), PASB brace (thoraco-lumbar and lumbar single curves), and Maguelone brace (kyphosis), Lapadula brace (kyphosis + scoliosis). Finally, we use the SpineCor brace for mild cases (up to a maximum of 30°).

With the exception of SpineCor, braces are custom-made following a CAD/CAM construction from laser body scanning. We fully comply with the SOSORT bracing guidelines which, in our view, is mandatory to obtain good results.

Do you continue to brace over 40°?

Yes. It is only a tradition to define the surgical threshold at 45°– 50°. We've published a couple of papers in which we have shown that 50% of curves between 45° and 60° can reach end of treatment below the surgical threshold. But treatment lasts on average five years and is demanding.

It's important to remember that surgery for scoliosis is fusing the spine, which means losing one of its functions—movement, in favor of another—stability. A young patient with a 45°– 60° curve has a visual trunk asymmetry, but usually nothing else. Generally, they don't have any other symptoms and to have a significant reduction of vital capacity you need a much worse curve (above 60°/70°).

Also, remember it is never a loss of time to first try conservative treatment, especially if the curve is below 60°. What we can guarantee with good bracing is an aesthetic result *(scoliosisjournal.com/content/4/1/18)* and in curves between 45° and 60°, we have an 8° to 10° curve reduction on average *(scoliosisjournal.com/content/4/S2/O50)*. This means that some patients remain stable or progress a little, but others "win the jackpot" and reduce their curve 15° to 20°. In the case of large, progressive curves, surgery must be considered. But in the case of curves that respond to bracing, surgery is usually avoided.

Would you still treat a patient conservatively if their curve is 60°?

Surgery is a treatment of the scoliosis curvature to prevent future problems that we know will happen almost for sure above 60°. Our approach is to ask the patient and family what they want to do. If they want to try conservative treatment, which is what we suggest, we have six months to see what can be achieved. If we are not able to achieve the outcome that the team desires, we tell the patient and family to consult with a surgeon in order to make an informed decision.

Surgery for scoliosis is not "quoad vitam" (to save life) but "quoad valetudinem" (to save quality of life). Surgical decisions must be agreed upon among the patient, family and the treating physician.

Can six months be an effective brace weaning period? What is your protocol?

The neuromotor system cannot react adequately to maintain the correction in six months. This could be good if you think of scoliosis only as a bone deformity. But when you recognize (as it is written in the literature) that there is also a postural component based on muscles and reaction to gravity force, you must give time to this system to react adequately, which in the end, will give better results. When good bone maturity is reached (Risser 3-4), we start going under 18 hours per day, which usually takes another 24 to 30 months before the brace is completely eliminated. In fact, the patients reduce the wearing time two hours every six months. So, gradually we reach the point when the ring apophysis (a measurement indicating that the spine is fully mature) usually closes at Risser 5. To avoid losing the correction, a gradual weaning is done in conjunction with exercises. This could explain why at the end of treatment, on average, we have an 8° to 9° curve reduction while others usually do not have improvements. We do not lose correction while weaning. This has been proven in another paper we published—scoliosisjournal.com/content/4/1/8.

SURGERY

When might you recommend surgery for a person with scoliosis?

We recommend surgery when problems are guaranteed into adulthood. This is an individual choice depending on Cobb degrees and many other factors. All patients must be well aware of risks on both sides — fusion versus conservative treatment for the rest of their life. Min Mehta, one of the most famous physicians dealing with scoliosis, never had her curve operated on and it was around 90°. Therefore, any individual choice is possible.

I think of how I would advise my own daughter if she had a large, significant thoracic curve with no other problems. If her curve was over 55/60° before starting any treatment, I would carefully discuss the possibility of fusion surgery because according to our study results, it is highly improbable that she could reduce her curve below 45°. Following some months of treatment without significant results, I would strongly suggest surgery, or I would suggest surgery immediately if she was not a candidate for bracing and her curve was above 60°. The final decision is made on a case-by-case basis, such as with a lumbar curve, which can be more dangerous and must be reduced. Or there may be other problems like significant imbalances, flatback, and so on that may require a surgical solution. All these factors must be taken into account with patients, their parents, and the multidisciplinary care team.

What are your guidelines when recommending surgery on a skeletally mature patient?

An adult scoliosis should only be operated on if they have significant symptoms, such as a scoliosis that is progressing, and specific exercises fail to stabilize it. Moreover, surgery should be considered when, despite conservative treatment, problems such as pain, impaired quality of life, diminished lung capacity, or a significant imbalance continue to persist. It must be clear to adult patients that if exercises succeed in stabilizing their curves, they must exercise for the rest of their life. If they cannot accept this, then surgery is preferable.

PART 6

Straight Talk

We cannot tell you the countless times we've heard parents say, "If I only knew" or more frustrated, "Why wasn't I told that?"

This section is devoted entirely to conversations with health care professionals offering you frank and thoughtful information on a wide variety of topics. Our work, both through the Curvy Girls' organization and throughout this book is simple — to arm you with knowledge to make the best decisions for your child's health care.

There is no reason any parent should echo the words, "If I only knew."

Information is power. Empower yourself!

DISCUSSIONS WITH ORTHOPEDISTS

James Barsi MD

Stony Brook University Hospital, NY

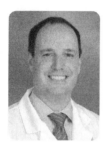

Dr. James Barsi is a Board-Certified Pediatric Orthopaedic Surgeon who specializes in complex scoliosis. He holds an appointment as a Clinical Associate Professor of Orthopaedic Surgery at Stony Brook University Hospital. He is a member of the Pediatric Orthopaedic Society of North America and the American Academy of Orthopaedic Surgeons. He has an active research focus on improving the lives of children with musculoskeletal conditions and has published numerous manuscripts and presented at national meetings. For more information, visit drjamesbarsi.com.

TREATMENT AND BRACING

Why is scoliosis a three-dimensional condition?

A scoliosis curve truly occurs in three dimensions. If you were to look at a spine from behind, there is a curve in the coronal or left to right direction. That is what is commonly measured on an X-ray using the Cobb angle. If we look at the spine from the side, there is often flattening of thoracic kyphosis or front to back curve of the spine. From an axial view, the rib protrusion that is seen during scoliosis screening tests comes from a rotation of the spine at the apex of the curve. By understanding how the curve behaves in these three planes, allows better brace design and surgical correction.

What is your treatment plan for a newly diagnosed patient?

A lot of factors come into play when developing an individualized treatment plan. That is truly the art of medicine combined with the science. When someone is diagnosed with scoliosis, I want to try to understand their risk of progression because that ultimately guides treatment. In general, curves below 25° are considered mild and are typically observed and prescribed scoliosis-specific physical therapy, such as the Schroth Method. Curves between 25°–50° would be prescribed a brace along with a script for physical therapy, as mentioned above. Curves greater than 50° are considered severe and at that magnitude I begin having a conversation regarding surgical options. These are generalizations though, and the treatment plan is tailored for each specific patient.

How many hours do you recommend that your patients wear a brace?

For adolescents with thoracic or thoracolumbar curves, I recommend 16 hours per day of brace wear. When I trained, the paradigm was 24 hours per day of brace wear. Recent studies have shown that brace compliance plays a large role in success at stabilizing the curve. That dose response effect (the more you wear a brace the better) plateaus at 16 hours. Statistically and clinically, there is no difference between 16 hours per day of brace wear and 24 hours per day of brace wear.

Is there a particular brace you find more effective?

We have come to realize that scoliosis is truly a three-dimensional curvature encompassing curvatures in the front and side planes, as well as a rotation in the axial plane. It makes sense to utilize a brace that addresses this complex nature of this condition. I have been using the Wood Chêneau Rigo (WCR) brace for the past five years and have been very happy with the results at stabilizing, and in some cases, even improving the spinal curve.

Under what circumstances would you only recommend a nighttime brace?

For isolated and flexible lumbar curves in adolescents with growth remaining, I would offer a nighttime brace. The mechanism of a nighttime brace is a hypercorrection of the curve by bending in the opposite direction. It is typically worn only at night because it is difficult if not impossible to wear the brace and function during the day.

Can a curve decrease while wearing a brace?

Traditionally, a brace was thought only to prevent progression; however, anecdotally and through recent studies, certain braces have shown the potential to correct some curves. We performed a research study at Stony Brook University trying to look into this and found that 45% of children who wore their WCR brace as recommended 16 hours per day and who performed a scoliosis-specific exercise program, such as the Schroth Method, at least five days per week had improvement of at least 5°.

What methods do you use to monitor remaining growth in your patients?

In general, girls stop growing around age 14, and boys stop growing around age 16. Traditionally, surgeons used the Risser sign to determine the end of skeletal growth. While easy to determine, there are several limitations with Risser. I use the Sanders criteria, which utilizes an X-ray of the left hand. We know that a hand has lots of bones and, therefore, lots of growth plates. Those growth plates close in a very predictable fashion. I can look at an X-ray of the hand and come up with Sanders score which has been shown to be more accurate than some of the other commonly utilized parameters.

What kind of follow-up is needed after bracing is complete?

While most small and moderate curves do not progress after skeletal maturity, some will. I typically follow patients two years after bracing.

Can curves continue to progress after skeletal maturity?

It really depends on the magnitude of the curve. Curves under about 30° will usually not progress. Curves greater than 50° will usually continue to increase, albeit at a slow rate estimated to be one to two degrees per year. The vast majority of curves between 30°–50° will not progress; however, a small percentage will. I believe even after skeletal maturity, it is important to keep up with a scoliosis-specific exercise program. For patients who demonstrated improvements in their curve by doing Schroth, I have found a rebound in curve magnitude when the exercises are not maintained.

Do you recommend surgery for skeletally mature patients at 50° curves?

A curve of 50° is what most would consider the threshold for considering surgery. I would start a conversation with the patient and family about surgery and discuss the risks and benefits of surgical intervention versus continued non-operative management. We know that statistically curves 50° and greater continue to progress—at a slow rate. From a functional issue, curves at 50° aren't usually associated with pain or compression of internal organs. That happens when curve magnitudes are higher. From a technical standpoint, surgical methods have advanced such that operating on a curve of 50° is equivalent to operating on a curve of 55°. As curves further increase in magnitude, they become stiffer though, and less correction would be expected unless maneuvers are performed during the operation to increase curve flexibility.

PAIN

Do you think physicians should ask if patients have pain?

I do. For newly diagnosed patients I want to make sure there is no other reason for scoliosis. For patients undergoing treatment, pain may suggest a brace not fitting properly or curve progression.

Under what circumstances would you order an MRI?

Usually I order an MRI for anyone undergoing surgical intervention as part of my pre-operative planning. We know that 20% of patients with early-onset scoliosis may have some type of abnormality on an MRI, so any infant or juvenile with a significant curve or curve progression, I would consider it. For adolescents, I order an MRI for anyone with atypical features: pain, fast progression, any positive neurologic exam finding, or any curve not appearing on X-ray as what I would think of as a traditional idiopathic curve.

PHYSICAL THERAPY

What role can scoliosis-specific exercises have in the treatment of scoliosis?

I am a big believer in a formal scoliosis-specific exercise program. First, I believe it empowers patients to take a direct role in their care. Second, I believe it increases compliance with bracing. My protocol is to follow patients every six months during their adolescent growth spurt. A therapist usually sees the patient one or two times per week. The constant encouragement by a healthcare professional helps the patient to wear the brace as recommended. Finally, I think scoliosis-specific exercises can play a role in increasing core strength, stabilizing and even improving curves. I always emphasize to patients that physical therapy is instructional. He or she goes there to learn the exercises; however, they must be continued at home to be effective.

SURGERY

What do you tell your patients to expect after surgery?

A lot of the nervousness surrounding surgery comes from the unexpected. I have an extensive family meeting with all of my patients who undergo surgery to go over my expectations during the post-operative period. We, of course, discuss the risks and benefits of the planned procedure but I also touch on post-operative pain control, which I think we have a much better understanding of now that we are using multi-modal pain medicine. That means we attack pain using different classes of medicine to better manage it.

When I trained, the average length of stay for scoliosis surgery was five to seven days. By making patients more comfortable, they are able to particpate in an accelerated physical therapy program which leads to earlier discharge. My average length of stay now is two to three days. Another common concern is whether or not the child will be able to return to their sports activities after surgery. I do restrict patients for a few months after surgery, but most patients will go back to the activities they love doing.

How do you decide what vertebrae to fuse?

The art of surgery is choosing appropriate levels. I want to choose enough of a construct length so that the spine is balanced and any curves above or below the fusion will not progress; however, I also want to preserve motion segments.

Is numbness and tingling near the incision normal after a year or more?

It is normal for the skin right next to the incision to feel strange or numb, sometimes permanently. In many cases, this is not very bothersome and the unpleasant sensation should get better over time but sensation may never return to normal. The legs or front of the chest shouldn't be numb.

Does having metal in your back prevent you from having an MRI?

No. Spinal implants now are usually a metal alloy. Some metals are more compatible than others. The metal can cause local distortion of the images. For example, I can order an MRI of the spine after instrumenting and the area directly around the screws and rods would be distorted slightly; however, the surrounding anatomy would still be visible. Imaging a distant part of the body, such as a knee or an ankle would be unaffected.

What kind of follow-up is recommended after surgery?

My typical protocol is to have patients come back for a wound check at two weeks. I see them back at the six-week, three-month, six month, one-year and two-year time points. I also like to see my fusion patients at five and ten years to check on how they are doing.

There is less long-term data regarding results and durability of the non-fusion procedures. For that reason, after the two-year follow-up visit, I ask patients to visit or send in X-rays at least annually to allow for early detection of any problem that might arise with the device. If they are doing well after two years, they graduate and only need to return if any issues arise.

Can a fused patient have an epidural?

It depends on where the fusion ends. However, most patients should still be able to have an epidural.

SCHOOL SCREENINGS

What do you recommend be done at a school screening?

A good screening test should consist of two parts. First, overall spinal balance should be assessed. This is typically done by examining the patient from behind and laying hands on the tops of the shoulders and then top of the pelvis. Any obliquity may suggest a curve present. Second, trunk rotation should be assessed. This is typically done with a device called a scoliometer. It is pressed against the spine and measures the rib prominence. Studies have shown that a scoliometer reading of seven degrees usually correlates to a curve under 20°.

Can someone pass a school-screening test and still have scoliosis?

Absolutely. Screening tests are not perfect. The goal of the screening test is first to find patients with mild to moderate curves whose progression may be altered by interventions, such as bracing or a scoliosis-specific exercise program. Patients with lumbar curves or patients on the heavier side tend to hide their curves better than those who are thinner or who have predominantly thoracic curves. If there is any concern, it is always better to see a provider who specializes in scoliosis.

A. Noelle Larson, MD

Mayo Clinic, MN

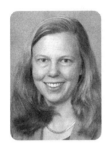

Dr. A. Noelle Larson is Associate Professor of Orthopedics, Director of Research for the Division of Pediatric Orthopedics and Scoliosis, and pediatric orthopaedic surgeon at the Mayo Clinic in Rochester, MN. Dr. Larson is certified by the American Board of Orthopaedic Surgery.

Dr. Larson has authored over 120 research publications in peer-reviewed journals. She co-directs the Minimize Implants Maximize Outcomes Randomized Clinical Trial and is the PI for a US surgeon-sponsored FDA Investigational Device Exemption study on fusionless scoliosis surgery, and is an active member of the Pediatric Spine Study Group and Harms Study Group.

Dr. Larson's clinical interests include spine deformity, early-onset scoliosis, and neuromuscular disease. Her practice includes intraoperative CT-guided navigation, 3D imaging techniques, and innovative approaches to complex spinal deformity. (mayoclinic.org)

What causes scoliosis?

The most common form of scoliosis is called idiopathic scoliosis, which means that we don't know what causes it. Scoliosis is a 3D curvature of the spine, primarily side-to-side. Scoliosis most commonly shows up in children during their rapid adolescent growth spurt. It can get worse rapidly as a child grows, and progression slows down or stops after the child is done growing. There may be genes that put some people at higher risk for scoliosis. Severe scoliosis is eight times more common in girls than boys. Some people think scoliosis is a growth plate problem. There is a growth plate above and below each vertebra of the spine. Growth plates that are compressed grow more slowly. Growth plates that have less pressure grow more quickly. So over the middle of a curve, the vertebra actually becomes wedged instead of square. This puts more uneven pressure over the growth plates, and the curve gets even worse.

Bracing, physical therapy, and some of the growth modulation strategies to treat scoliosis are based on the principle of unloading the compressed growth plates in the spine. There is a lot of research going on trying to figure out which patients are at most risk for the curve getting worse and how best to prevent this.

TREATMENT AND BRACING

What is your treatment plan for newly diagnosed patients?

Once a child is diagnosed with scoliosis, I meet with the family to discuss treatment options including observation, bracing and physical therapy. Children who are still growing and who have curves between 10° and 20° require follow-up visits every six months with X-rays to monitor for progression. When their curves progress over 20° they become a candidate for bracing. For curves 40°– 60°, surgery can be considered. However, this number depends to some extent on how much growth the child has remaining and, thus, how much rapid curve progression is likely.

It's important that all the girls get the information and emotional support that they need. For that reason, all the girls who visit my office are provided with a Curvy Girls' flyer. I also always provide my phone number as a resource if more questions arise. Parents and patients should always feel free to seek a second opinion, because these are important life changing decisions, and each family has to do what they need to do to feel comfortable with the treatment plan.

Is bracing effective?

A prospective randomized study published in the New England Journal of Medicine, which is one of the top medical journals, found that bracing was effective. This was a $5 million dollar study performed at 25 sites around the US. A rigid TLSO (thoracolumbosacral orthosis) or a Boston-style brace was used in this study. All patients wore a temperature monitor in the brace, so that the number of hours of wear was objectively recorded. For patients who wore their brace 13 hours a day, 28% of the children required scoliosis surgery compared to 52% if no brace was used. If patients wore their braces 18 hours per day as prescribed, surgery rates were even lower, closer to 10%. Also, if an X-ray taken with the brace on showed good correction, there was a better chance of the brace working.

What is your protocol for a first in-brace X-ray?

The first thing I require is a standing in-brace X-ray on date of brace delivery with the straps as tight as possible. The child doesn't have to start out with the straps that tight at home, but I would like to see what the brace can do when it is really tight.

Since this is usually an emotional visit, as children face the reality of wearing a brace, I set time aside to give families an opportunity to ask questions about bracing and to discuss the plan on how to start brace wear.

After the brace fitting, I provide patients with a copy of the X-ray in the brace versus out of the brace which was taken at the previous visit. This is a visual cue of the power of the brace and hopefully may provide encouragement for patients through the tough weeks ahead of getting used to wearing the brace.

Is there a particular brace you find more effective than others?

Yes. I would recommend a rigid brace that achieves 30-50% correction of the curve when an X-ray is taken while wearing the brace. Further, the brace should be comfortable and discrete enough so that the child can actually wear the brace. There is the most evidence to support a TLSO or Boston-type brace. There was a very high-quality study (prospective randomized controlled trial) of the TLSO which was published in the New England Journal of Medicine. This is one of the top journals in all of medicine, and it is quite rare for an orthopedic study to be published in this journal. This article showed that a TLSO resulted in a lower rate of significant curve progression compared to no treatment. I am also interested in the concept of the Rigo Chêneau-type brace, which is extensively used in Europe. To my knowledge, there is only one retrospective study comparing the Rigo Chêneau-type brace to a standard TLSO, which did show better outcomes with the Rigo Chêneau brace, but there were only 13 patients in the study with a Rigo Chêneau brace and 95 with a TLSO. Further high-quality prospective studies are needed on this topic.

What kind of in-brace correction do you expect to see?

I aim for 40% correction in brace. For example, a curve that measures 30° on an X-ray out of the brace will measure 18° for an X-ray in the brace. It is important to have an X-ray taken in the brace on at least one occasion to ensure that the brace is holding the spine in a corrected position.

How many hours a day do you recommend your patient wear their brace?

There is a dose response between hours of brace wear and curve progression. More hours in the brace result in decreased risk of curve progression. So it is a continuum. Maximum benefit is likely 18 to 20 hours a day.

I recommend 16-20 hours a day for high risk patients (younger with curves over 30°). Children who are close to being done growing may do fine with part-time brace wear or even nighttime brace wear only. I think it is important for children to remove the brace for physical activities each day and for special events. Some children are opposed to wearing the brace to school. The school day is a long period of time where there is not much physical activity (except for gym class), so it is a logical time to wear the brace. On the other hand, some patients are not comfortable with this. It is possible to succeed with brace treatment by wearing the brace evenings/weekends/nighttime if the child is very dedicated to this program.

How quickly can a curve progress?

During rapid growth, curves can progress up to 20° in one year.

What impact can the scoliosis-specific exercises have on a person with scoliosis?

Schroth or scoliosis-specific exercises can alleviate back pain and improve quality of life. It makes sense to me that training the muscles to support the spine could function like a brace or be used as a complement to bracing to prevent progression of the curve.

There have not yet been high quality studies with greater than two-year follow-up showing that Schroth improves the curve or prevents curve progression long-term. However, I have seen individual patients with excellent results from scoliosis-specific exercises often in conjunction with bracing.

Can scoliosis-specific exercises be beneficial for a skeletally mature spine?

Yes. It is very important to focus on scoliosis-specific exercises when the brace is being discontinued so that muscles can take over for the work that the brace was doing. Building strong abdominal and back muscles may help prevent back pain and promote long-term good health. Scoliosis-specific exercises require ongoing time and commitment on the part of the patient and family.

Is there a curve limit to prescribing a brace?

I am almost always happy to prescribe a brace. It gives families time to consider their options before making an important decision. Very large curves—those greater than 70°—likely do not benefit from bracing, particularly if the curve is rigid and there is not much correction in the brace.

SURGERY

At what degree do you discuss surgery?

I will strongly recommend surgery for curves over 60°, particularly if there has been progression after the child is done growing. Many surgeons recommend surgery at 50°, and this is the U.S. standard of care presently. Surgery may be a reasonable option for curves between 40° to 60° based on the child's growth remaining, the surgical approach, and patient and family preferences.

Why are there discrepancies among surgeons as to when a patient can return to activities/sports following spinal fusion surgery?

Return to sports after scoliosis surgery **has not been** well-studied in orthopedics, so there are no clear evidence-based guidelines. It certainly deserves more research. Similar to bracing, where it is hard to standardize patient brace wear, it is also hard to standardize activity levels. Further, it is such a rare occurrence to have a problem that many patients would need to be studied in order to figure out when it is best to return to sports following spine surgery. It may depend on other factors such as bone quality, amount of scoliosis correction, length of fusion, and type of activity. Therefore, it is very reasonable to restrict sports for three to six months after spinal fusion.

In my practice for fusion surgery, patients can swim and use an exercise bicycle or elliptical starting four weeks after surgery. Patients are cleared for many sports by three months. Other surgeons allow return to activities after surgery as tolerated. This is primarily a judgment call and families should be involved in the decision-making. In some instances, if the child is done growing, it may be possible to delay spine fusion until the child has completed high level competition. For instance, few people play tackle football after high school or college.

Are there circumstances in which a surgeon might delay return to activities?

For collision sports such as motocross, football, or ice hockey, some surgeons would restrict participation for six to 12 months or even forever. Fusions that extend into the lumbar spine, very large curves, or poor bone quality noted during the surgery would be other reasons that surgeons may delay clearing a child to return to sports.

Can body weight affect fusion hardware long term?

Very overweight patients (BMI percentile > 95%) have a higher rate of infection following scoliosis fusion surgery (up to 7x higher). They also may be at increased risk for implant pullout at the top or bottom of construct, particularly if the child has rounding of the back or kyphosis.

Underweight children may have more prominent implants. This has been associated with increased infection risk, particularly in young children and those with other medical problems.

In adulthood, obesity is a risk factor for back pain and other serious medical problems.

Michael G. Vitale MD, MPH

Pediatric Orthopaedics, NYP Hospital, NY

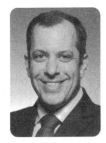

Dr. Michael G. Vitale *is a world-renowned specialist in the non-operative and operative treatment of complex pediatric scoliosis and spinal disorders, performing approximately 200 scoliosis procedures every year – half of which are in children less than 10 years of age. Dr. Vitale's surgical practice leverages specialized multidisciplinary teams to optimize care of adolescents with scoliosis, and uses innovative treatments for younger children with scoliosis, including* magnetic spine lengthening rods *("MAGEC"), and non-fusion procedures such as anterior vertebral tethering for juvenile scoliosis. He also has a special interest in the conservative management of scoliosis and leads a best-in-class team of* Schroth scoliosis therapists, Rigo Chêneau-style bracing *experts, and cast technicians with extensive experience at Mehta casting. Dr. Vitale is consistently recognized as one of America's Top Doctors by Castle Connolly, and has been named among the top 50 physicians providing scoliosis care in the US by Becker's Spine Review. (pediatricsoliosis.com)*

What is your treatment philosophy?

I see myself as the conductor or gardener in the care process. My role is to get the right resources together and to present the available data in a way that families can make the best decision for them. Few things are absolutely black and white in this space and patient preferences matter. I have worked to create the very best care team for patients both under conservative care and for those who have surgery. It makes a big difference when the people on the team are 100% focused and committed only to taking the very best care of kids with scoliosis. When we need to do surgery, it's my obligation to make sure that the surgery is done at the highest level, in the safest manner and also maximizing the patient's and family's experience. Over many years of a high-volume practice, we have been able to build protocols that are continually optimized to take the best care of our patients.

What is your treatment plan for a newly diagnosed AIS patient?

The degree of curvature determines the plan of care for a newly diagnosed AIS patient. Often if the curve is 10-25°, which is considered a mild scoliosis, the recommendation will be observation with follow up

X-rays and supplemental vitamin D and calcium until full growth has been reached.

For a curve of 25–40° in a skeletally immature patient, the recommendation would be for bracing and close follow-up to include both in- and out-of-brace X-rays. We would also recommend scoliosis-specific physical therapy, such as Schroth therapy and supplemental vitamin D and calcium.

What led you to recommend vitamin D and calcium supplements?

There have been two very well-done studies showing efficacy of vitamin D supplementation in decreasing curve progression in AIS. Moreover, many pediatricians recommend vitamin D and calcium to their patients routinely as part of good bone health. In addition, the dosing recommended is in a range where it is extremely unlikely that there could be any side effects.

What is your brace of preference?

We recommend the Rigo Chêneau brace. Both biomechanical and clinical research, including that of our group, suggests that 3-dimensional braces like the Rigo brace achieve better 3-dimensional in-brace correction and result in lower rates of curve progression. We are working to achieve consensus on this point through an SRS/SOSORT sponsored best practice guideline.

Do you prefer an in-brace X-ray the day the child receives their brace or do you wait several weeks for their body to adjust to the brace?

Our preference is to take the in-brace X-rays 4–6 weeks after the brace was originally received.

How many hours do you recommend your patient wear their brace daily?

Our standard recommendation is that they wear the braces 18 hours/day but we often try to fine tune this recommendation based on the perceived risk of progression (related to skeletal maturity and curve size).

Why is there a discrepancy among orthopedic spine surgeons regarding the number of hours for brace wear?

Again, the evidence base supporting these recommendations is not so strong and orthopaedic surgeons interpret this in different ways and have different feelings about the "costs" of bracing (psychosocial and activity modification during adolescence).

There seems to be a lack of consensus in the field as to the required out-of-brace hours prior to follow-up X-rays. What is your approach?

That's true. Here, we instruct patients to be out of the brace at least 12 and up to 24 hours before an out of brace X-ray. I think this is the sweet spot where there is no real risk related to being out of the brace for a bit but still where its likely we will get the most honest X-rays.

What methods do you use to monitor remaining growth in your patients?

We use the Sanders Maturity Scale (SMS) which involves doing a series of hand X-rays to monitor patient's growth. In our view, multiple studies including our own have shown this to be more accurate than other staging systems.

Can you explain Sanders scoring system versus Risser staging?

Both the SMS and the Risser correlate with menarche. However, when looking at growth with AIS, the SMS is a more precise indicator for correlating to the rapid phase of growth, thus, the greatest risk of curve progression. Use of Risser alone will result in "bad" decisions about bracing one out of five times.

If a child is initially diagnosed with a 50°curve and has growth remaining, what would your treatment plan be?

It really depends on the skeletal maturity of the child and the curve location. For children who are Sanders 2 or above with structural thoracic curves but non-structural lumbar curves, surgery is generally recommended. In almost all cases, a selective thoracic fusion will stop progression and even result in spontaneous resolution of the lumbar curve without lumbar fusion which is really ideal. On the other hand, if a patient already has a large lumbar curve and is well balanced, I'll often attempt "aggressive conservative care" (Schroth, vit D, RCB). In much younger kids, we sometimes consider growing strategies including MAGEC, anterior tether or Shilla, though this is a complicated discussion and decision.

PHYSIOTHERAPY SCOLIOSIS SPECIFIC EXERCISES

What made you decide to expand the conservative care component of your practice?

Several years ago, we made a commitment to incorporate PSSE and 3D bracing into our treatment protocol. The research and literature had become, in my opinion, compelling enough to invest in these programs and to change our protocols.

We are all on a journey to be better at what we do. For me, my mission is to take the very best care possible of children with scoliosis and to help to continually improve how we do that. This is where clinical research and quality improvement intersect and I'm proud of the progress we have made in the last couple decades. I love the book "Upstream" which talks about solving problems before they happen. We all need to do better at being holistic doctors in this space, not just surgeons. I'm lucky to be surrounded by skilled and dedicated team members including nurses, PAs, orthotists and physical therapists who make us better.

How do you introduce PSSE to your families?

Most of my patients come having heard about PSSE but even for those who do not, its intuitive that it might help. I review the literature including the 4-5 randomized trials in this space. It's been my observation that patients who participate in PSSE are more engaged in their own care and more compliant in the brace.

You offer comprehensive care with a multidisciplinary approach. Tell us about that?

We now have a better appreciation of optimal bracing (3D braces like the Rigo-style brace with attention to in-brace X-rays and compliance monitoring), appropriate indications and dosing of bracing, the role of scoliosis physical therapy and possibly vitamin D supplementation. These are some of the elements of "best practice" but they are changing and I anticipate/hope they will continue to change over time.

SURGERY

Why is there a difference of opinion among surgeons as to when patients require spinal fusion surgery?

The "book" answer is most generally agreed to be curves 45–50°. There is some difference of opinion because the natural history of curves in this range is not fully understood. The evidence seems to show that almost all curves in this range or higher in children who are growing will progress but things are less clear in children as they end growth and enter young adulthood. To me, the decision needs to be a shared decision with patients and families incorporating their preferences around other issues besides curve size including cosmetic appearance, concerns about the possibility of surgery in the future, and concerns about the possibility of more involved surgeries if the curve progresses or extends further distally.

Can body weight affect fusion hardware long term?

We often recommend that our patients gain five pounds before their scheduled spinal fusion. It is common for patients to lose a little weight during and after spinal surgery. Optimal nutrition is a vital component to the healing process after spinal surgery. In the very smallest children, hardware can be prominent and there are some "tricks" to help with this. The main issue with heavier kids is the increased risk of wound problems and infection. We often use a plastic surgeon for obese kids and use special types of dressings.

PATIENT EDUCATION

Annually you provide a non-operative education seminar for medical professionals and patients. Why was this important?

We have published best practices for conservative scoliosis management based on a thorough review of the literature and consensus among experts. There is still too much variability in how patients are treated and this implies that some patients are not getting the very best treatment. Our educational offerings are a way of moving the bell curve and helping everyone understand the best practices for the care of children with scoliosis.

Tell us about your book, **Scoliosis: A Guide for Children and Their Families.**

I really wanted to have a book out there with medical information aimed at patients and their families. So many of my patients wanted to share their stories. Amber Sentell, my coauthor did an amazing job helping with this. Many patients have told me that they find it very valuable.

Laurence E. Mermelstein MD

Long Island Spine Specialists, Long Island, NY

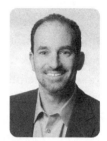

Dr. **Laurence Mermelstein** *is a Board-Certified Orthopedic Surgeon whose clinical practice places an emphasis on pediatric and adult scoliosis and deformities, adult degenerative conditions, and minimally invasive surgical techniques. As the first surgeon on Long Island, New York to perform the Posterolateral Endoscopic Discectomy procedure, he continues to be on the forefront of surgical technology. He has lectured extensively at national and international meetings regarding Spinal Biomechanics, Spinal Instrumentation and Intraoperative Neurophysiological Monitoring. He has volunteered his expertise internationally in caring for children with severe complex spinal deformities and conditions through his involvement with SpineHope, a 501(c)(3) nonprofit organization based in Austin, TX. (www.lispine.com)*

DOCTOR-PATIENT RELATIONSHIP

What should parents look for in an orthopedic surgeon when their child has scoliosis?

I would recommend that parents look for an orthopedic spine/pediatric orthopedic surgeon who has experience with pediatric scoliosis surgery. The surgeon should be familiar with ALL types of surgical approaches so that he can discuss ALL different options with equal experience. Preferably, the surgeon should have a practice specializing in spine surgery (as opposed to a surgeon taking care of a mix of spine and non-spinal issues).

I understand you speak directly to your young patients, rather than addressing your remarks to the parents. Can you tell us why you think that is important?

The kids are the patients here. They need to take ownership of the decisions, whether they want to or not. Of course, the heavy lifting when it comes to decisions is still done between the parents and myself, but it is very important that the kids feel involved. Otherwise, I might as well be doing veterinary surgery. When the kids have involvement in the decisions, they do not feel as powerless and they are involved in their recovery—and results are better.

What do you recommend to a parent/patient when they don't feel that their medical provider is listening or addressing their concerns?

I would ask them if there was another time or forum outside of the traditional office visit where they could communicate. Email has been helpful in getting extra time and answers. Phone conferences after hours are helpful as well. Sometimes the doctor can feel very rushed and strained in the middle of clinic hours. They may be able to listen and respond better in another format. If that doesn't work, you may need to seek answers elsewhere.

Is it possible that although it's called "adolescent" scoliosis that it may have existed undetected years before? Is it just the adolescent growth spurt that makes scoliosis more apparent?

By definition, idiopathic scoliosis is not present at birth. Again, by definition, it is first detected in kids, 10 to 16 years of age. If the curve is seen before 10 years of age, it is termed "juvenile" or "early onset" idiopathic scoliosis. The earlier that the curve presents, the more likely the curve will progress. It is certainly possible that smaller curves in younger patients go undetected until adolescence. It is with the rapid growth acceleration that occurs with puberty that the magnitudes of these curves sometimes increase rapidly.

What do you do when a child complains of pain?

If a child complains about having pain I will assess the problem to make sure nothing more serious is going on. Processes like infections or tumors can cause pain and a reactive (secondary) scoliosis. If there is no evidence for another cause of pain than a child might benefit from some scoliosis-specific exercises, such as the Schroth Method. If pain continues, an MRI may be indicated.

BRACING

Do you have a brace of preference?

Over the last eight years, we have been recommending the WCR (Woods Chêneau Rigo) modification of the Rigo Chêneau bracing system. Studies comparing the success of different bracing systems have demonstrated improved curve correction and lower incidence of progression to surgery in the WCR when compared to older systems, such as the Boston brace, which I had used previously.

I also continue to use the Charleston bending brace, a nighttime only brace, in select children with select curves. This has obvious advantages with respect to compliance.

Why is there a discrepancy among orthopedic spine surgeons regarding the number of hours for brace wear (16 hours versus 23 hours)?

Research has shown that the more time a child spends in the brace, the better. The efficacy is "dose" (time) dependent. To my knowledge, there is no "threshold" time above which it is not helpful or even counter-productive. My experience is that, in kids, we shoot for twenty-three hours a day, realizing the actual time will be much less, accounting for bathing, swimming, sports, and gym class.

If a child had a 20° curve, would you begin bracing as an early intervention?

Not usually. I probably would just continue to monitor that child. I don't like to put a child in a brace any earlier than I have to. If the patient is 17 years old and four years post-menarche, there are no reasons to brace. However, if there is evidence of family history of scoliosis, I might be more aggressive. If I have an eight-year-old child who has a rather stiff curve, and whose mother and grandmother had surgery on their scoliosis, I would intervene with bracing sooner.

When do you decide your patient needs full-time bracing?

I usually will start full-time bracing when the curve reaches 25° and the child still has a lot of growth remaining. If for some reason I'm not sure about the growth remaining, I will send them for a bone age X-ray. The benefit of the hand/wrist film is that it gives you a different perspective on their bone age.

What factors do you use to determine when bracing is nearing its end?

Bracing is usually completed when a patient is skeletally mature. This is determined in a number of ways, some more complicated than others. Simple methods are a patient's menstrual history (in girls, of course), their height in comparison to their parents/older siblings, iliac crest growth plates (Risser sign) that is easily seen on X-rays of spine. If there is any debate, a "bone age" using X-rays of the left hand can be obtained. The growth plates of the hand are compared to an "atlas" of typical children of a similar "age" and skeletal maturity is assessed.

The simplest way, if I have the data, is to look at the growth curve, which I can develop from my chart of height in the office. If a child has not grown in two consecutive visits, and other factors as above are in agreement, we can discuss a weaning protocol. This is less true in boys who can have late, unpredictable growth accelerations.

Do you implement a weaning phase for your patients?
To be clear, just because a child has been diligent at wearing a brace and they hit milestones that say she is skeletally mature, doesn't mean they discontinue the brace and all is well. It is not uncommon for a child with a curve, which has been well controlled in the brace to demonstrate progression of their curves after they stop the brace (even though they are skeletally mature).

Depending on the type of brace and the numbers of hours the brace is being worn, we slowly increase the hours out of the brace and recheck X-rays at subsequent visits. If a curve progresses with decreasing brace wear, we stop the weaning and maintain the bracing time. Sometimes this means we are continuing bracing well after growth has ceased. Depending on the magnitude of the curve when kids reach skeletal maturity, curves can continue to progress as "young adults" when bracing is eventually stopped. In these cases, we discuss surgery to arrest the progression (and correct the curve).

Can curves continue to progress post-bracing?
Yes. Curves can progress after a brace is worn and growth ceases. I wish I could tell you why this happens in some patients and not in others. Many times, it has to do with the degree the curve winds up in after growth ends. Curves that are close to 40° and above have a higher likelihood of progression into adulthood, than curves less than 30°. That is why surgery is recommended for these larger curves; they do tend to progress, albeit at a slower rate than during puberty.

Do you recommend PSSE as part of your treatment plan?
Yes, I do recommend these specific exercises as part of a holistic approach to scoliosis management. This approach to scoliosis treatment

was developed by Katharina Schroth and further popularized by her daughter Christa. Born in Germany in the late 1800s, Katharina Schroth had scoliosis that was unsuccessfully treated with bracing. She developed her own breathing technique and exercises to manage her scoliosis. It is only recently in the last 10 years that this program has been used by physical therapists in the US. The Schroth therapist focuses on elongating and derotating the scoliotic or kyphotic spine, in an effort to stop/slow curve progression and prevent further spinal curvature. A treatment session typically lasts 45 minutes and encompasses hands-on stretching, passive positioning and active breathing techniques. There are a relatively small number of therapists who provide this treatment, as it requires additional certification and significantly more time. Studies are underway to determine if this approach is able to arrest or reverse the progression of scoliosis.

SURGERY

What accounts for differences among surgeons regarding the degree to surgically correct scoliosis?

There is no absolute consensus regarding surgical indications for scoliosis. Indications for surgery are not based on degrees alone, although there is a general number of about 45°, give or take. The goals for surgery are correction, obviously, but equally important is to arrest progression. Not all 40° to 45° curves have the same risk. Thoracic curves are more likely to progress and the younger the patient the more likely surgery is suggested. A curve that is imbalanced is more likely to require surgery. Indications for adult scoliosis surgery are completely different, and more likely to require surgery for pain at a lesser degree magnitude. Different surgeons will be more or less aggressive and they each have their own reasons. It is the same for ALL types of orthopedic surgeries, arthroscopy to joint replacements.

What is an anterior fusion?

Fusion surgery for scoliosis performed from the side is called an "anterior fusion." It is most frequently used for primarily lumbar curves. In this surgery, the entire disc is removed and the anterior ligaments released. This may allow for a better correction. Bone graft is put directly in between the vertebrae in the disc spaces. Usually, anterior instrumentation is put on the side of the vertebrae holding the correction until fusion is achieved. The advantage of this is that fewer vertebrae can be fused, especially lower down in the spine. Also, a selective lumbar fusion can be done, which is much less surgery. Lumbar and thoracic curves cannot be addressed with this approach at the same time. A separate surgical incision would be needed to address a thoracic curve at the same time; therefore, it is not usually done in double major curves (unless the curves are so stiff that they need an "anterior release"). Disadvantages are that the instrumentation fixation may not be as good anteriorly, as it is with pedicle screws posteriorly.

What is an intra-operative monitoring system?

Intra-operative spinal cord monitoring (IOM) has become the gold standard for monitoring the function of the spinal cord during scoliosis correction surgery. Over the last 15+ years, the motor and sensory function of the spinal cord can be continuously monitored in real time during the surgery. Electrodes are placed on the patient's skull and in various muscles in the abdomen and legs. Impulses are sent to the brain and recorded in the muscles and vice versa. Any intra-operative maneuvers or corrections that may impair spinal cord function can be reversed in a timely fashion, thereby, minimizing post-operative deficits. Prior to the advent of IOM, a "wake-up test" was performed after the correction maneuvers and before the wound was closed. The patient was woken up while still on their stomachs during the surgery. If they had trouble moving their feet and legs, a spinal cord injury may be detected.

When making a decision about surgery for a child, what should parents look for in a hospital?

The hospital has to be used to handling complex spinal procedures in the operating room with respect to anesthesia, instrumentation, and equipment. Cell Saver® blood scavenging needs to be available. Spinal cord intra-operative monitoring (IOM) needs to be available with staff experienced in these cases. The hospital needs to have a post-operative monitored care environment (ICU or "stepdown") that is comfortable taking care of spinal surgery patients. It is always helpful to be close to home so that post-operative complications can be handled in a timely fashion. It is nice that the parents can stay with the child as much as they desire (although I do recommend they get some quality sleep at some point!).

RECOVERY

While in the hospital, how will a parent be able to assess if their child's pain is being managed effectively?

The patient should be able to roll from side to side and be able to get out of bed without a severe amount of pain. Pain cannot be completely eliminated, nor should this be the goal. If a patient is over-medicated, they will be overly sedated, and unable to participate in physical therapy and walking.

How soon after a child's spinal surgery do you recommend getting out of bed?

The next day.

When do you allow your patients to return to gym/sport activities?

Full healing from scoliosis surgery requires full healing of a spinal fusion. Typically, this takes at least four to six months, sometimes longer. It also depends on the amount of surgery (how long a fusion) the patient had, as well as the type of sport. For any impact activity or activities requiring twisting and lifting, I prefer to wait at least nine months before clearing for activity.

Are there any activities long term that could cause pain after spinal fusion surgery?

Running, tennis, golf, gymnastics, etc.

Generally, after a child has healed 100% from surgery, most activities should be pain-free. If a child has a significant amount of lumbar spine fused, she may feel stiff or restricted in their mobility due to loss of motion in the lower back. Because of this, if a child has undergone a significant lumbar fusion, I counsel against activities such as gymnastics and certain types of dancing that require a significant range of motion. Otherwise, I allow kids to go back to almost all types of sports except contact sports (football, rugby).

Nigel Price MD, FAAOS, FAAP
Children's Mercy Hospital, MO

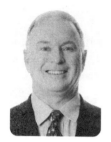

Dr. Nigel Price has been a spine surgeon practicing at Children's Mercy Hospital in Kansas City, Missouri for 25 years. He is the Spine Section Chief and an Associate Professor of Orthopedic Surgery at the University of Missouri, Kansas City. He is the Pediatric Orthopedic Fellowship Director and the Surgical Telemedicine Director. Dr. Price has a particular interest in early onset scoliosis management and the non-operative treatment of scoliosis and has helped to advance these interests through his affiliations with the Scoliosis Research Society and SOSORT. He is currently the chair of the Non-Operative Committee of the SRS. (childmercy.org)

BRACE TREATMENT

Do you have a brace of preference?

The brace that I am most familiar with, and have prescribed for over 25 years, is the Boston Brace and the newer version of the brace with 3D features. I have preferred this brace because my orthotist and I are most proficient with it and it is well tolerated by patients. It was also the most common worn brace in the BrAIST study of which we as an institution were the largest contributor of patients. However, a year ago my main orthotist and I attended the Rigo course and now have a second 3D brace, the Rigo 3D which we are prescribing.

What percentage of correction do you want to see from a new brace?

This is somewhat based on each patient's individual characteristics. Age, maturity, magnitude and type of curve all factor into expectations. A younger female patient with a thoracolumbar or lumbar curve and a thin body habitus may get over 50% correction. An older male patient with a larger thoracic curve may not get more than 10%-20%. There are other considerations such as achieving a balanced spine in the brace in both front and side planes. Patients sometimes don't tolerate overly aggressive bracing to achieve larger in-brace correction.

When do you order an in-brace X-ray?

I always wait for the patient to wean into bracing for at least six weeks of full-time use before I get an X-ray. I find that this minimizes the guesswork of whether there is an issue with compliance or brace design if the in-brace radiograph is not what we hope to see.

Some surgeons request patients out of their brace 3-5 days prior to follow-up X-ray? What is your opinion on this?

I am familiar with the out-of-brace protocol but I don't follow this. I prefer to consider the in-brace radiograph as a tool that the orthotist and I can use to determine optimum fit and correction. I was trained to do the X-ray in brace for that reason and I still do it this way for most patients. Occasionally, I will do an out-of-brace X-ray.

Does the size of the curve make a difference on the bracing hours you recommend?

A little. Some patients come to me with curves in the 40° range. If the patient is young, there is a greater chance of the patient progressing to need surgery. So, I am inclined to suggest, at least initially, up to 22 hours a day in the brace. I have seen some instances where a patient started with a curve over 40° and ended up with a smaller curve after weaning out of the brace at maturity.

Do you recommend the PSSE to your patients?

I send many of my patients for Schroth exercises. I believe that the Schroth scoliosis exercises complement the brace treatment. I also educate all my patients across the scoliosis spectrum, including mild curves that are under the threshold for bracing and severe curves in patients who don't want surgery about these excercises.

Have you ever recommended children wear two types of braces—one for daytime and one for nighttime?

I have not routinely done this. It is more expensive and most insurance companies would deny coverage in my experience. For some curve patterns it could be advantageous, so I am not opposed to it and I have had some patients do it.

Do you wean your patients from bracing?

Yes, I do wean patients gradually out of the brace. I think that I have fewer patients experiencing back pain and I do think that they are more likely to rebound quickly and past the original Cobb angle prior to bracing. As they wean out of brace, I encourage them to do flexibility exercises and core strengthening exercises. I typically encourage scoliosis-specific physical therapy exercises, such as the Schroth Method.

SURGERY

At what degree do you begin to discuss surgery?

I do have a conversation with the family at 50°. I prefer to call it educating the family about the options. There are other options emerging such as non-fusion procedures, so I make sure that the family knows that a definitive fusion and instrumentation is not the only option. I also reassure them that depending on the patient's age, maturity and concerns that the patient may have about the effect the curve is having, there can be a very large window in which to do surgery. I have many patients who are observed with curves over 50° and are doing fine. They sometimes "age out" of my adolescent practice and continue to be observed by my adult scoliosis colleagues.

Do you recommend PSSE for pre- and post-op spinal fusion patients?

I do. I refer all patients for physical therapy pre-op, during their hospital stay and post-op. I think that they mobilize better, have better balance and possibly less pain.

If a child has a curve over 50° with growth remaining and a parent would like to attempt 3D bracing in conjunction with scoliosis-specific exercises, would you support their decision?

Honestly, this is a longshot. For a young patient with a Risser sign of 0 (ideally less than one or two) who is premenarchal or just post-menarchal, I would explain that there is no great harm in this but there is no strong support in the literature. If the brace is tolerated with a curve magnitude over 50°, I will consider a trial. There are also new federal FDA non-fusion operations that are discussed such as Tethering and ApiFix as alternatives.

Craig Eberson, MD
University Orthopedics, RI

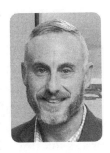

Dr. Craig Eberson graduated from the University of Pennsylvania with a degree in Neural Systems, and attended medical school at The University of Medicine and Dentistry of New Jersey-Robert Wood Johnson Medical School (now Rutgers) in New Jersey, his home state. After his Residency and an Orthopedic Trauma Fellowship at Brown University/Rhode Island Hospital, he served as the Dorothy and Bryant Edwards Fellow in Pediatric Orthopedics and Scoliosis at the Texas Scottish Rite Hospital for Children, in Dallas, Texas.

Dr. Eberson returned to Rhode Island to join the faculty at Brown University Alpert School of Medicine, where he currently serves as the Chief of the Division of Pediatric Orthopedics and Scoliosis, as well as the Program Director of the Orthopedic Surgery Residency. His practice and research interests include spinal deformity surgery, neuromuscular disease, and pediatric orthopedic trauma. He has authored more than 60 peer-reviewed publications and multiple book chapters. (universityorthopedics.com)

TREATMENT AND BRACING

What are some commonly asked questions from parents after they learn their child has scoliosis?

Parents are concerned that something they did—like letting their daughter carry a backpack full of heavy textbooks—caused the scoliosis. I reassure them that there is no evidence that mattresses, backpacks, doing your homework in bed, sports, or chronic texting cause scoliosis. They are also concerned if their child may have to avoid any sports. I do not limit sports participation in any child with scoliosis.

Do you have a brace of preference?

I like to use the Providence brace, since it can be worn only at night, but for larger curves, or for patients who don't tolerate that brace, I will also use a Boston Brace or WCR brace.

What percentage of correction do you want to see from a new brace?

For a Boston about 50%, for Providence about 85% or greater.

How many hours do you recommend your patient wear their brace?
Providence eight hours; Boston 16-18.

Have you ever recommended children wear two types of braces—one for daytime and one for nighttime? If yes, was it beneficial?
Yes, for kids with larger curves (over 35°- 40°), or for kids who progress in a Providence brace, I will use a Boston during the day and a Providence at night. The braces fit and work slightly differently, and the kids seem to tolerate the braces better. This gives them a full bracing regimen—Providence plus additional brace time in Boston. For the rare child who cannot sleep in the Providence brace, I have also used Boston braces full time (16-18 hours)

What methods do you use to monitor growth remaining in your patients?
There are several methods I use to monitor growth remaining, such asheight, menstrual status, pelvic growth plate (Risser sign), and Sanders stage /bone age from a hand film.

What can cause a curve to progress rapidly?
A rapid curve could be triggered by an underlying neurologic pathology (tumor, tethered cord, syrinx, Chiari malformation, etc.), or a connective tissue disorder (Marfan, Ehlers Danlos).

Do you suggest scoliosis-specific exercises such as the Schroth Method?
I offer Schroth to all of my patients that are interested. The patients need to be old enough and committed enough to comply with the exercise regimen, and be motivated to do their exercises at home. I think the research is not conclusive at this point, but I feel that there are definitely patients who will benefit from Schroth, often in addition to bracing. The skeletally mature patient with a visually objectionable thoracolumbar curve is often able to learn to stand and move in a more "balanced" fashion with Schroth.

SURGERY

At what curve degree do you first discuss surgery?
Usually over 50°.

Can patients who are very thin have more sensitivity or discomfort in their backs after surgery?

Occasionally, they will be bothered by the profile of a screw or crosslink.

What is a crosslink?

A crosslink is a device used to literally link the two rods together to make the whole construct stronger. Sometimes they are prominent. With the advent of stronger rods and screws, some surgeons will leave them out to avoid irritation.

When can a post-op patient resume sports activity?

This depends upon the activity and the extent of the fusion, but generally kids can go back to their sports by 6 months after surgery. Some sports (gymnastics, ballet) that require significant flexibility may be difficult to do after extensive surgery, but most common sports (baseball, tennis, golf, soccer, swimming, cheer, etc) are fine. Contact sports (football, lacrosse) are at the discretion of the surgeon.

Fusionless Surgeries

Over the years, there have been exciting new techniques available for families when contemplating a surgical intervention for their child's scoliosis—fusionless surgeries. We hope the information we provide will better prepare you when discussing this topic with your surgeon.

VERTEBRAL BODY TETHERING

Joshua Pahys, MD
Shriners Hospital for Children, PA

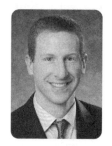

Dr. Joshua Pahys is an orthopaedic surgeon for Shriners Hospitals for Children — Philadelphia and is board certified by the American Board of Orthopaedic Surgery. He received an undergraduate degree in biology from Johns Hopkins University and earned a medical degree from Jefferson Medical College.

Dr. Pahys completed his residency in orthopaedic surgery at Albert Einstein Medical Center and a fellowship in adult and pediatric spine at Washington University in St. Louis, Missouri. Dr. Pahys is a member of the Scoliosis Research Society and a fellow of the American Academy of Orthopaedic Surgeons. He is also a member of the Harms Study Group, Children's Spine Study Group, Pediatric Cervical Spine Study Group, and a board member of the Philadelphia Orthopaedic Society. He serves as the residency and fellowship director for Shriners Hospitals for Children — Philadelphia. He is active in research and has authored numerous publications, book chapters and presentations. (shrinershospitals4children.org)

What is Vertebral Body Tethering (VBT) for scoliosis?

VBT is a growth modulation surgery. Screws are placed on the anterior (front) of the spine along the convex (outside) portion of the spinal curvature. The screws are connected to one another with a flexible cord. The cord is tightened between each screw to compress the convex portion of the curve and impart some correction on the curve. This one-sided compression of the growth plates in the vertebrae slows the growth of the vertebrae on the outside of the curve (convex portion), allowing the concave (inside) portion to "grow straighter" with time. In short, the outside of the curve becomes tethered, and the inside of the curve "grows faster" relative to the outside. This asymmetric growth ideally results in continued curve correction with time after the surgery in skeletally immature patients.

When was this procedure first performed?

The first published case report was by Dr. Lenke in 2010. We started performing this procedure at Shriners Hospitals for Children – Philadelphia in 2011.

Is this approved for use in the United States?

VBT was approved as a "Humanitarian Use Device" by the Food and Drug Administration (FDA) in August 2019. The approval came after several years of collaboration with Shriners Hospitals for Children – Philadelphia, the FDA, and the medical device company. The approval was based on a retrospective review of 57 patients who underwent VBT at Shriners Hospital for Children – Philadelphia and were followed to skeletal maturity.

The FDA-approved indications for VBT are for skeletally immature patients with idiopathic scoliosis curves from 35° to 65° in the thoracic and/or thoracolumbar spine. To be eligible for this surgery, patients need to fit this criteria when recommended/offered by their surgeon. The surgeon is also required to undergo training with the device prior to their first case. Multicenter prospective studies are now underway to further study the procedure as well as the short- and long-term outcomes.

What qualifications should a parent look for when selecting a surgeon to perform VBT?

Surgeon experience and comfort level with anterior thoracic surgery and/or VBT is recommended. Some surgeons will visit VBT centers to learn/observe the procedure prior to performing the surgery themselves which is also ideal, but not mandatory.

Who is a good candidate for this procedure?

Our indications for VBT are:
1. Curves 40° to 65° have to reduce to less than 35° on bending films. We have found that larger, stiffer curves have a higher failure rate with VBT.

2. Skeletally immature (growth remaining) defined as a Risser 0-1 (seen on the pelvis) and/or a Sanders bone age of 5 or less (obtained with a hand film) are eligible. We do not perform VBT (a growth modulation procedure) on skeletally mature patients (patients with little to no growth remaining).
3. Ideally females should be premenarchal or within 6 months of their first menses.
4. The typical minimum age for VBT is 10 years. Patients under 10 years of age generally have too much growth remaining, and thus have a higher chance for overcorrection.

Are adults or skeletally mature adolescents candidates for VBT?

The FDA mandated that the procedure only be performed on "skeletally immature patients with idiopathic scoliosis" and lists "skeletal maturity" as a contraindication. However, some centers have performed the procedure on mature patients as physician-directed off label use. Thus, if a particular physician believes this procedure will work on a mature patient, they are not prohibited from performing it and can do so at their discretion, despite FDA guidelines against it.

The principle of VBT relies on growth modulation (getting the spine to "grow straight"). Thus, if there is no growth remaining, a growth modulation procedure would not be indicated.

Philly Shriners' concern is that the tether may hold the spine in a straighter position for a period of time. However, if the vertebrae do not modulate, or "grow straighter," we are very concerned that the rope will inevitably break and the spine will regress back to its previous deformity. The patient would then require a fusion; the procedure that may have been recommended at the onset for a mature patient with progressive scoliosis.

What about a child with growing rods?

We have not recommended VBT for patients with growing rods, as there is a concern the spine may be too stiff and not flexible enough for VBT to reliably work. Further, the new FDA indications prohibit VBT on patients who have had prior spine surgery.

Does the Scoliosis Research Society provide guidelines on VBT?

The SRS has provided an informational statement on VBT, but the Society cannot formally permit or prohibit a surgeon from performing a particular procedure. The Society can provide data to its members and a forum for discussion on possible indications and contraindications for the treatment of scoliosis. The SRS informational statement regarding tethering in mature patients reads: *"While research in animals may provide future opportunities for VBT in adult spinal deformity, it is important to emphasize that no data has been published to date confirming the safety or efficacy of this technique in adults."*

How is VBT different than spinal fusion surgery?

Spinal fusion is most often performed from a posterior (back) approach, whereas VBT is performed via an anterior approach. With spinal fusion, the fused area of the spine is fused/immobilized permanently. This prevents curve progression, but may limit motion in the area of the construct. VBT acts to prevent curve progression, but ideally retains more motion in the operative portion of the spine as the screws are connected via a flexible cord, compared to a rigid rod (fusion). Lastly, a spine is fused as straight as possible during surgery. With VBT, the spine is left with some residual curve to allow for continued correction of the curve with growth after surgery. Our results show that spinal fusion has achieved better results for clinical outcomes (shoulder imbalance, rib prominence reduction, and trunk shift) compared to VBT. This is because the surgeon can straighten the spine as much as possible with a fusion at the time of surgery. With VBT, we can only partially straighten the spine during surgery, and the remainder corrects with patient growth. This further correction with growth can be variable amongst patients.

Does VBT correct scoliosis rotation?

VBT has been shown to have some correction of rotation and rib prominence, but typically much less than with spinal fusion. The correction of a rib prominence is typically between 50-75% with a spinal fusion and 25-50% with VBT. Fusion corrects the curvature and rotation of the spine at the time of surgery and locks that into place. The correction of rotation is much more variable and less predictable in VBT where correction relies on remaining growth. We have seen cases where the curvature corrects over time, but the rib prominence does not. For this reason, a large rib prominence (>25°) is a relative (but not absolute) contraindication for VBT.

Do you address this with families interested in this procedure?

We have extensive discussions with our families who are considering VBT versus spinal fusion. We caution our families/patients considering VBT that the cosmetic outcome (rib prominence, trunk and shoulder asymmetry) is much more variable with VBT compared to spinal fusion. If these are significant concerns for the patient/family, VBT may not be the right procedure for them.

If the rotation is not corrected, could the curve progress after a year?

Not likely. The typical reason for curve progression a year after surgery is the tether has ruptured between two screws. This occurs when the growth plates of these two vertebrae did not modulate, or "grow straight," and thus, the tether alone was maintaining the correction the entire time. If the vertebrae do not "grow straight" and the tether is under constant tension it can eventually rupture and the curve regresses in this one area. A curve that has a significant amount of rotation prior to surgery may be an indication of an underlying more aggressive deformity in which the tether may not be strong enough to overcome.

What are the pros and cons when considering VBT surgery?

Pros:
1. Potentially maintaining spinal motion post-op
2. Earlier return to activities/sports (6 weeks vs. 12 weeks)
3. Smaller incisions

Cons:
1. Higher reoperation rate compared to post-spinal fusion (10-15% VBT vs. 5-10% fusion)
2. Involves thoracic surgery where the surgeon typically has to deflate and re-inflate the lung to have access to the spine
3. Less reliable cosmetic outcome (rib prominence, shoulder imbalance)
4. No long-term data to date

Can you tell us about reoperation?

The reoperation rate for VBT is approximately 10-15%. We do not know the long-term implications of a tether, as we have only been following patients for 8 years.

The most common reason for reoperation is overcorrection, requiring the tether rope to be cut. The tether can also rupture and the deformity can regress. We have seen this most commonly 1-2 years after the surgery when the patient has matured. If the curve remains stable and only regresses slightly, no reoperation is required. If the curvature continues to worsen, and the patient is skeletally mature, a fusion may be required.

What are the chances a person would need another fusion later in life?

We have studied spinal fusion patients for over 40 years and know there is an approximately 5-10% chance over their lifetime that they will require another operation.

What kind of follow-up is needed after VBT?

It is important to have a clinical visit at least once a year and an X-ray every 6 months while the patient is growing. The surgeon can monitor for any significant overcorrection, as well as ensure the tether remains intact.

Are there any sports restrictions after this procedure?

No. We recommend to limit bending, lifting, twisting (BLT) for 3-4 weeks post-op to allow the incisions to heal. After this time, the patients are allowed to slowly return to activities as tolerated.

What impact does increased body mass have on VBT outcomes?

Complications rates—rope breakages are higher and success rates lower for VBT in obese patients, which the Center of Disease Control (CDC) defines as a Body Mass Index (BMI) at or above the 95th percentile for children and teens of the same age and sex.

Anything VBT patients need to watch for down the road?

If a patient experiences progressive and persistent back and/or leg pain, they should contact their surgeon or local physician for a check-up.

APIFIX

Nigel Price MD, FAAOS, FAAP

Children's Mercy Hospital, MO

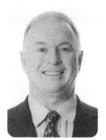

Dr. Nigel Price is currently a Professor of Orthopedic Surgery at the University of Missouri, Kansas City. He is the Chief of the Spine Section at Children's Mercy Hospital. He has been practicing pediatric orthopedic surgery with an emphasis on early onset scoliosis and adolescent scoliosis for over 27 years in the Midwest. Dr. Price has helped to bring non-fusion techniques to Children's Mercy which was one of the first US centers to have IRB approval for two new devices, ApiFix and VBT. He continues to promote early detection and non-operative spine care and when indicated non-fusion or fusion techniques for spinal deformity.

What is ApiFix?

ApiFix's *Minimally Invasive Deformity Correction (MID-C) System* is a posterior dynamic scoliosis correction system that enables surgeons to perform a novel treatment providing permanent curve correction while retaining spine flexibility with a least invasive approach. FDA approval via a Humanitarian Device Exemption (HDE) was received in August 2019.

Does the device placement change depending on where the primary curve is located?

The ApiFix device is surgically placed unilaterally on the concave side of the spinal curve. The device is available in various lengths (sizes) to treat Lenke type 1 (thoracic) curves and Lenke type 5 (thoracolumbar and lumbar) curves.

How long does this procedure take?

An ApiFix surgery typically lasts 90-120 minutes.

How do you achieve correction without fusion?

The unique ApiFix approach provides a viable alternative to unsuccessful bracing before considering spinal fusion for many patients as the least invasive spine deformity correction option versus vertebral body tethering (VBT) and spinal fusion. The MID-C System acts as an "internal brace" with motion-preserving polyaxial joints and a patented unidirectional, self-adjusting rod mechanism allowing additional post-operative correction over time; it is ultimately removable.

What qualifications or training is required for a surgeon to perform this surgery?

Patients and families should be sure to consult with pediatric spine surgeons who focus on treating adolescent idiopathic scoliosis and related conditions. The ApiFix system is implanted via a posterior approach familiar to all pediatric spine surgeons. The surgeon must also have IRB (Institutional Review Board) approval before implanting the device.

What are the guidelines for this procedure?

The ApiFix MID-C System is indicated for use in patients with adolescent idiopathic scoliosis (AIS) for treatment of single curves classified as Lenke 1 (thoracic major curve) or Lenke 5 (thoracolumbar/lumbar major curve), having a Cobb angle of 35° to 60° which reduces to less than or equal to 30° on lateral side-bending radiographs, and thoracic kyphosis less than 55° as measured from T5 to T12. Use of the MID-C System in patients with curves of lower magnitudes (less than 40°) is based on the risk for curve progression.

What is the expected recovery?

The ApiFix device is implanted via a unilateral posterior procedure where patient recovery is relatively pain-free and is measured in days, not months. Children are discharged from the hospital in one-to-two days and return to school or work in one-to-two weeks.

Does the ApiFix procedure correct the scoliosis rotation?

The ApiFix procedure is able to restore shoulder balance and address rib hump in curves that have up to 20° of rotation and are flexible on lateral bending. Curves with rotation greater than 20° tend to be more structural in nature (not as flexible) and, thus, these patients are not good candidates for a successful ApiFix outcome.

If the rotation is unable to be corrected, can this cause the curve to progress?

Mild rotation (<20°) can typically be corrected or addressed allowing for adequate curve correction with minimal risk of post-surgical curve progression.

How is this procedure different from VBT?

The ApiFix procedure utilizes a standard posterior approach to the spine which is a familiar approach to pediatric spine surgeons. Vertebral Body Tethering may require an additional surgeon in the operating room to access the spine through the chest. During the anterior approach, the patient's lung on that side of the chest is temporarily deflated and a chest tube may need to be inserted to help re-inflate the lung and may require a stay in the ICU after surgery. None of this is necessary with the ApiFix procedure.

What role, if any, does PSSE have in treatment and/or recovery?

Exercises before surgery to increase spinal flexibility (especially after extended brace wearing) are always encouraged but not required. These exercises after surgery are not a necessary part of the treatment or recovery plan but are recommended to help with body alignment after curve correction.

Is a child with growing rods a candidate for ApiFix?

Growing rods (magnetically controlled growing rods) are typically used for treating early onset scoliosis (EOS). The ApiFix system is intended for treating adolescent idiopathic scoliosis and therefore a child treated with growing rods is not a candidate for ApiFix.

What is the likelihood a patient would need fusion later in life?

A typical AIS patient successfully treated with ApiFix whose resultant curve after surgery is <30° should never need to have fusion surgery.

What possible complications can occur from this procedure?

There is always the risk of complications with any surgical procedure which can be device-related (implant breakage, loosening, migration or other mechanical failure and inadequate curve correction) or non-device-related (infection, foreign body reaction, adverse reaction to anesthesia, etc.)

Have there been re-operations?

The ApiFix system has been in clinical use for treating patients with progressive scoliosis outside the United States since 2012 leading up to FDA approval of the technology in 2019. Over the course of this clinical use, there have been re-operations for a variety of reasons including:

i) removal of the implant; ii) replacement of the implant with another ApiFix system; iii) removal of the implant and conversion to fusion or another technology.

The clinical data from the historical clinical use of the ApiFix system support the reasonable assurance of safety and probable benefit of the MID-C System when used in accordance with the indications for use.

What kind of follow-up is required after surgery?

Expect a standard follow-up protocol: post-operatively, 6 months and annually, thereafter.

Are there any sports restrictions after this procedure?

Patients implanted with the ApiFix system should not participate in contact or high demand sports such as weightlifting, tumbling, gymnastics, rowing, or other high-risk activities as this could lead to loosening of the implant.

How long do these restrictions last?

These restrictions would be in place indefinitely or until implants are removed.

To be a candidate for removal the patient must have had the device for a minimum of three years and maintained a 25° curve. Hopefully this is an acceptable trade-off given the longer-term prospects of an active and normal lifestyle.

What might be a cause for procedure failure?

Proper patient selection (adhering to the indications for use) is of paramount importance in ensuring the success of the ApiFix procedure along with proper implant selection and placement during the surgical procedure.

How does BMI (body mass index) impact the procedure?

There is not a defined BMI limitation for the ApiFix procedure but surgeon discretion on the basis of BMI, patient activity level, bone quality, and other factors is necessary. Generally speaking, there is evidence in the literature of a significant increase in complications in patients with BMI≥35 following spine surgery, with that rate further increasing with BMI≥40.

Connecting the Dots

POTS – EDS – SCOLIOSIS

On a number of occasions, we have witnessed children who have experienced symptoms that appeared to be unrelated to scoliosis, leaving physicians baffled. After much delay and frustration, these children were ultimately diagnosed with syndromes that can, in fact, be co-occurring with scoliosis. By including a section on both POTS (Postural Orthostatic Tachycardia Syndrome) and EDS (Ehlers-Danlos Syndrome), we hope to help the parents of the small percentage of children to connect the dots sooner and receive appropriate treatment.

UNDERSTANDING POTS & EDS

Phil Fischer, MD

Mayo Clinic, MN

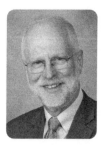

Dr. Phil Fischer graduated from medical school at the University of California, Irvine, and completed a pediatric residency at the University of Utah. For more than two decades, he has been caring for adolescents with chronic fatigue and chronic pain at the Mayo Clinic in Rochester, Minnesota, where he is professor of pediatrics. He also helps out with the admissions process at the Mayo Clinic Alix School of Medicine where it has been his great pleasure to welcome one of his recovered former POTS patients as a medical student. He has authored more than 200 medical publications and co-edited a textbook produced through two editions by the American Academy of Pediatrics. *(mayoclinic.org)*

What is Postural Orthostatic Tachycardia Syndrome (POTS)?

POTS is a disorder of the autonomic (involuntary) nervous system by which the body doesn't regulate blood flow adequately, especially in response to gravity. As blood tubes (vessels) fail to tighten, blood pools in legs when upright; this leaves less blood in the circulation and causes dizziness, even though the heart beats faster to try to compensate. Related involuntary nervous system abnormalities lead many POTS patients to have trouble with their stomachs and intestines, too, as well as difficulty regulating body temperature.

Are you born with POTS?

No. It usually develops around the time of early adolescence as the child enters puberty.

Who is more at risk for developing this syndrome?

POTS usually occurs in high achievers—those adolescents who did extremely well in school and extra-curricular activities prior to getting sick. Some families seem more prone to POTS than others. People with stretchy joints (hypermobility) also seem more prone to develop POTS. Adults can also develop POTS later in life.

What are the symptoms of this condition?

Almost everyone with POTS has dizziness when standing, along with chronic fatigue. About two-thirds of POTS patients have headache or abdominal pain. A majority of POTS patients have nausea or intestinal irregularity. Many have trouble thinking clearly ("brain fog").

Can POTS have a psychological impact?

Yes. It's is very hard for these kids to deal with this disorder. POTS makes teenagers feel tired all the time. It makes them dizzy when they stand up. It makes school and social situations challenging, and it makes some adolescents drop out of life.

Is this a lifelong condition?

POTS is miserable during these years but the vast majority of adolescents who develop POTS can (and do) fully recover and return to normal life activities. Many adults with later onset POTS also improve or even recover.

How is POTS diagnosed?

The diagnosis is based on: 1) chronically feeling worse when upright (usually with dizziness) and better when lying down, and 2) having an excessive increase in heart rate when switching from lying to standing. Essentially always, there are symptoms every day, not just intermittently.

What is the process for making a diagnosis?

A doctor or other medical provider needs to understand the story to see if there really is long-term trouble being upright (orthostatic intolerance). He or she needs to make sure there is not a different medical diagnosis (anemia or thyroid trouble or something else) masquerading as POTS. And, testing must confirm a sustained increase in heart rate (pulse) of at least 40 beats per minute (30 for adults) going from lying calmly (or better yet, being tilted on a formal tilt table test) to standing totally still for ten minutes.

What is the treatment protocol?

Patients should build their blood volume by greatly increasing fluid and salt intake. They should strengthen their muscles and nerves with daily aerobic exercise. They should maximize the positive input from their minds with cognitive behavioral therapy. And, most benefit from medication to facilitate blood flow (usually a beta blocker or midodrine) to treat other associated symptoms/conditions.

What is Ehlers-Danlos Syndrome?

EDS is a collection of hypermobility syndromes. Patients have stretchy joints. Some have severe enough trouble that joints fall out of place. Very rare patients with one form of EDS can even have swelling in their blood vessels. Some EDS can be confirmed with genetic testing (of specific genes related to the manufacture of cartilage and other connective tissues). The names and labels for EDS keep changing, but hypermobility is at the core, and it is only a minority of patients who have severe activity-limiting problems.

What are the symptoms?

Usually not many at all – just stretchy joints and, sometimes, joint pains.

Do you have to be hypermobile or extremely flexible to have EDS?

Hypermobility is at the core of the various forms of EDS.

Is there a link with POTS and EDS?

Patients with hypermobility seem also to have "stretchier" blood vessels and, thus, to be more prone to POTS with challenges keeping blood vessels "tight" when standing up.

Are there any correlations between these conditions and scoliosis?

Yes. Scoliosis is more common with EDS than in other people (though most people with scoliosis do not have EDS). Lots of POTS patients have scoliosis, but it is not clear that scoliosis is actually more common in POTS patients than in other people without POTS.

How do you treat EDS?

Usually, all that is needed is to strengthen the muscles around bothersome stretchy joints, and physical therapists can help guide this. Some EDS patients develop chronic pain and can benefit from chronic pain medication and cognitive behavioral therapy. Only in a rare few, would orthopedic surgery be needed.

Is EDS a lifelong condition or is this something you can outgrow?

EDS persists, but joint hyper-flexibility can improve with aging.

Low-Dose Radiation

Learn about low-dose X-ray exams with EOS imaging.

EOS IMAGING SYSTEM

Dana Goldy, RT

Dana Goldy has been working as a radiology technologist for more than 28 years, graduating from San Diego Mesa College in 1992. She is licensed by both the state of California (C.R.T.) and the American Registry of Radiologic Technologists (A.R.R.T.). She spent the majority of her career specializing in pediatric trauma and orthopedic imaging before transitioning into a supervisory role.

Since 2011, Dana has worked as the Senior Application Specialist for EOS imaging performing training for technologists and physicians around the globe. She has spent extensive time helping to develop training programs and educational tools on the EOS imaging system. (eosimaging.com)

What is EOS imaging?

EOS imaging offers a low-dose, weight-bearing X-ray system. It can simultaneously capture full spine or full body, frontal and lateral (side view) images of the skeletal system in a standing or sitting position using significantly less radiation than a traditional X-ray or CT-scan.

With EOS, two dimensional (2D) and three-dimensional (3D) orthopedic images can be produced to assist doctors with the diagnosis, treatment and management of medical conditions like scoliosis.

How is EOS different from standard X-ray?

EOS provides, in one scan, a front and side image of the patient's full spine or entire body. EOS images avoid a traditional X-ray process called stitching, where images are combined to create a single front (or side) image. Research has shown stitching may result in a measurement error of a Cobb angle,[1] which EOS avoids by providing accurate one-to-one images for physicians to make precise measurements.

EOS also has the capability to evaluate scoliosis in three-dimensions. Because the spine is a 3D structure, having this additional level of detail can help physicians further understand scoliosis and guide treatment.

Perhaps most importantly, EOS is low-dose. That means the patient's EOS imaging procedure and effective dose of radiation will be As Low As Reasonably Achievable (ALARA).

How much is the radiation dose from an EOS exam?

One of the biggest concern parents have with repeated X-ray imaging for scoliosis is radiation exposure. An EOS exam delivers 50%[2] to 85%[3] less radiation than traditional X-ray systems and 95%[4] less dose than computed tomography (CT) scans.

Reducing radiation dose is particularly beneficial for children with scoliosis requiring frequent imaging. The Micro Dose feature further reduces radiation exposure, offering full spine images that are equivalent to only a week's worth of natural radiation, or roughly a 90% reduction compared to a standard X-ray exam.[5]

Can you tell us more about Micro Dose?

Micro Dose is a unique setting only available through EOS imaging. The setting further reduces dose by slightly reducing image quality, yet still provides an image with enough resolution to measure the Cobb angle and other scoliosis parameters. The exam is typically reserved for follow-up imaging exams (monitoring) and can significantly reduce radiation exposure—beyond what's possible even through EOS—to further minimize any potential long-term harm from X-rays.

How is 3D assessment with EOS being used today?

EOS 3D measurements provide physicians with accurate parameters of the patient's spine. 3D measurements remove traditional 2D measurement bias, allowing for more confident diagnosis, treatment planning and confirmation of treatments. For conservative measures, such as bracing, EOS 3D measurements can precisely evaluate how effective the treatment has progressed.

Sometimes when conservative treatments fail to provide enough correction, surgery may be an option. EOS 3D measurements can be used by surgeons to plan the operation, using 3D models to simulate what type of rods and instrumentation are best to restore the patient's spinal alignment. After treatment, 3D measurements can be used to confirm the success of conservative care or a surgical operation.

Leading healthcare organizations use EOS 3D measurements in clinical research to validate existing strategies and prove new concepts. EOS 3D measurements provide precise data sets and are captured in a weight-bearing position (standing), where traditional 3D measurements from other imaging sources, such an MRI or CT scan, are typically collected while the patient is lying down.

What should you expect from the exam?
The patient will stand in the EOS cabin while the X-ray is taken. The exam uses two very fine X-ray beams that are capable of simultaneously capturing both frontal and lateral images of the patient. The EOS system can image the entire spine in less than 20 seconds. The total exam time takes about 4 minutes including preparation and patient positioning.

What is the EOSedge system?
In 2020, EOS imaging introduced a new imaging platform called EOSedge. The system is based on the design of the EOS system, yet delivers exciting new technological advancements, such as higher image resolution and new Flex Dose™ technology.

Flex Dose™ technology allows for dose modulation along the patient's body reducing dose in less demanding areas and increasing dose in important areas. This technology expands on EOS imaging's low-dose and Micro Dose technologies that aim to reduce radiation exposure.

In addition, the EOSedge system's photon counting detection technology delivers high-resolution X-ray images that allow doctors to diagnose and evaluate scoliosis. It's the first X-ray-based system to incorporate this type of technology. Similar to the EOS system, 3D measurements can be generated from EOSedge X-ray images.

How can a parent request EOS imaging?
EOS imaging is available at many large healthcare institutions and children's hospitals in the United States and countries around the world. When you meet with your physician, make sure to ask whether or not your child will be receiving an EOS exam. If it's a follow-up appointment, be sure to ask whether or not your child will be receiving an EOS

Micro Dose exam, which further reduces the dose. In some instances, you may be able to drive to the nearest EOS location before your doctor's appointment to have an EOS imaging exam performed.

Does health insurance cover this type of imaging?

An EOS exam is billed under standard insurance X-ray insurance codes that are commonly covered by most insurance plans.

How can our readers find out where the nearest EOS is located?

Readers can find the closest EOS facility through the EOS imaging website: www.eos-imaging.us

References

[1] Supakul, Nucharin, et al. "Diagnostic Errors from Digital Stitching of Scoliosis Images – the Importance of Evaluating the Source Images Prior to Making a Final Diagnosis." Pediatric Radiology, vol. 42, no. 5, 2011, pp. 584–598., doi:10.1007/s00247-011-2293-y.

[2] Diagnostic imaging of spinal deformities: reducing patient's radiation dose with a new slot-scanning x-ray imager. Deschenes S et al. Spine. 2010

[3] Comparison of radiation dose, patient comfort and financial break-even of standard digital radiography and a novel biplanar low-dose x-ray system for upright full-length lower limb and whole spine radiography. Dietrich TJ et al. Skeletal Radiol. 2013

[4] Ionizing radiation doses during lower limb torsion and anteversion measurements by EOS stereoradiography and computed tomography. Delin C, et al. Eur J Radiol. 2013

[5] EOS Micro Dose protocol for the radiological follow-up of adolescent idiopathic scoliosis. Ilharreborde B. et al. Eur Spine J. 2015

PART 7

Psychological Support and Guidance

Robin Stoltz, Licensed Clinical Social Worker

Learning from Adversity: Twist of Fate

The current generation of parents have often been labeled as "helicopter" or "lawnmower" parents in their desire to protect their kids. "Helicopter" parents are notorious for hovering over their children to monitor and be prepared to step in to every aspect of a child's life and experience; "lawnmower" parents stand ready to "mow down" any obstacles that may challenge their child's level of comfort or perceived skills.

This very act of overprotecting from disappointment and pain, however, actually yields the opposite effect of obstructing healthy child development and readiness for assuming adult roles and tasks. By not allowing our children to experience and work through problems on their own and at their own pace, they cannot learn necessary skills to work through life challenges. We are inadvertently telling them, *"You are not equipped to deal with this; I need to do it for you because you are not capable."* As a result, we are making them dependent upon us to solve their problems, and worse, hindering the development of their self-esteem and confidence to take on challenges. As children seek to differentiate themselves from this dependency, they come face-to-face with self-doubt about their competency and their future. ABC News reported in November 2019 that colleges are struggling with soaring demand in their counseling centers. "On some campuses, the number of students seeking treatment has nearly doubled over the last five years."

Since a sense of confidence and success can only emerge from experience, what we really need to do is allow our children to master their own challenges and build their own coping tool box. The only way we enable our children to do that is by pulling back against our impulses to help and allowing our children with our support to experience disappointment, frustration, and even failure—even as it makes us cringe with our own worries and fears. Our job as parents is to help our children learn to navigate all the challenges of pre-adolescence and adolescence and not play interference.

The insult of a diagnosis of scoliosis offers the affected child and family an ironic "twist of fate": Its appearance at critical points of development, and the subsequent journey, offers many opportunities for life lessons that will prove beneficial to our children as they face other life challenges into their adulthood—while also affording parents their own feelings of success and even freedom as we seek to pursue later life enjoyment.

I recall the day my child began middle school wearing her new brace. Feeling totally helpless, I worried that my daughter would be teased and her heart would be broken because she would see that kids can be mean. I worried she wouldn't know how to respond if kids or teachers said something that made her feel uncomfortable. I felt self-conscious for her. I wanted to be with her to protect her from hurt and shame. But I did nothing. I held my tongue and then held my breath awaiting her return.

> **Resilience is a trait that all parents need to teach their children, but one which requires the parent to allow the child to experience the pain of disappointment.**

Because the scoliosis journey corresponds with several phases of development, it presents our children with opportunities to try out many new coping strategies and skills that they can build upon over the time of their maturation into adulthood. Coping skills are taught, learned, and experienced. I like to say to my kids, "Stuff happens; now we have to figure out how to deal with it." After all, how can you learn to "bounce back" if you've never experienced a setback? Most of all, the scoliosis journey can be an experience where they might witness themselves overcoming challenges and become more capable and self-confident than they were before scoliosis, but only if you let them. Time and again, we see through Curvy Girls that many children emerge stronger, more confident, and more focused. No one wishes their child to be diagnosed with a condition like scoliosis. But if there's a hopeful prospect to this difficult life challenge, it may be this opportunity for personal growth.

While you had no control over the diagnosis, you can control how you respond to it! According to Dr. Kenneth Ginsburg, a well-known physician of adolescent medicine, professor and author of "Raising Kids to Thrive," you can be a "Lighthouse Parent" —

> *Visible from the shoreline as a stable light or beacon. They should make sure their children don't crash against the rocks, yet allow them to ride the waves even if they get a little choppy sometimes.*

In many Curvy Girls' parent support meetings, I challenge parents to ask themselves, "*Who is this solution for and who will feel better as a result?*" We must learn the skill of sitting with our own discomfort and not fixing the problem or interrupting the experience, so that your child *can discover their own way of coping and their own voice.*

Communication 101

For parents of kids with scoliosis, figuring out when to be firm or lenient can be a challenge during adolescence. My husband, Mike, and I struggled mightily with when and how firmly to discipline. Sometimes it is difficult to remain consistent when teens become adept at finding our vulnerabilities and pushing those buttons, especially when one of the buttons is guilt.

We found ourselves questioning our own judgment: *"Was I too hard on her? After all, maybe she's feeling bad today about herself because of the brace. Did someone say something to make her feel bad? But then again, she mouthed off to me. If I ignore this, it gives her the message that the behavior is acceptable. When should we give her leeway?"*

We didn't think it would be a good message to be easier on our daughter for behaviors that were not acceptable, simply because she has scoliosis. We always had to ask ourselves what it was that we were disciplining—frustration with her body image or poor behavior. It was the unacceptable behavior that we had to discipline, while finding a way to help her to talk through her feelings.

GETTING TEENS TO TALK

Here are some hints:

- *Ask open-ended questions, where the response can't be given in one word answers, such as, "yes," "no," or "good."*

Examples to start conversations are, "I was wondering what you thought about _____" or "Tell me about _____" —with enthusiastic interest— interspersed with reflective statements like, "That's really interesting" and "I am really impressed with how you think about that."

- *Spend time together outside of the house (walking, shopping).*

Often these activities allow opportunities for conversation. Because you, as an adult, are in control in your house (or so it seems), taking your teen off-grounds levels the playing field. Leah was more inclined to talk when we weren't at home. You'll be surprised by the new information you might learn about your teen's life and you may not even have to ask! Just listen.

- *Talk about things that might interest teens.*

When a teen feels that you are really tuned in and interested in hearing them talk about their interests, even if they are not similar to your own, they may be more likely to discuss other elements of their experiences. Plus, these conversations can give you insight to their emerging values and sense of judgement, which "sets the table" for important future discussions.

- *Try not to take your child's display of frustration personally.*

After everything we do for our children as part of our parent job, it's hard to not take lashing out or negative behavior (especially when aimed at us) personally. In service, allowing children the space to experience their feelings, we often need to check our own feelings/responses, such as hurt and/or anger at the door. If, however, a behavior is inappropriate, then a parent has to address it by saying something like "That's not acceptable."

Be creative in your approach; consider humor to help break a mood but NOT sarcasm. And then be ready to have a sincere conversation when your child is able to chat.

- *If none of that works, there's always counseling.*

My husband and I are both psychotherapists. Leah has watched me treat adolescents and, as a young child, would sneak into my office area to try to meet them. I'd smile to myself, certain that this would pave the way for her teenagehood. Yet when it was her turn to be a teen, speaking with me about her experiences was out of the question. She told me, "I don't do feelings." Silly me! But when she got so angry one night that she slammed my bedroom door breaking the mirror, it was time for intervention beyond what we could provide. She was making it clear that she needed help with all she was shouldering and all we needed to do was to acknowledge her distress and give her potential outlets.

Ironically, the drive to her counseling sessions proved to be a time when she taught me about the importance of a "neutral" gear: In the neutral setting of the car, she talked about her day and shared other thoughts. If I wasn't too intrusive (read: bite my tongue), she would even share more.

That being said, you need to know your own child and how much connection and intervention is too much. But, as a rule, if over a period of time your child is withdrawing from social contact and activities, or crying with any frequency, it's time to intervene.

Seeking Support

Our experience has been that once a child/teen is involved with a group of peers who understand what they are dealing with, any sense of despair they may experience from feeling different will diminish. Contact your nearest Curvy Girls' support group and help your child get involved. CG peer groups are located internationally and are there to help support you through this journey. Online support for girls is also provided through the Curvy Girls' website at curvygirlsscoliosis.com.

If, however, you find that your child/teen needs more than peer support, do not be afraid to seek professional advice. Seeking help does not imply that you did something wrong or failed your child. Nor does it mean that something is wrong with your child. The purpose of seeking professional advice is to help guide you and your child through difficult challenges in life. Common themes that the experience of scoliosis may complicate are body image issues, learning problems, and family circumstances.

Choosing a Mental Health Professional

If your child would benefit from speaking with a mental health professional and you live in the United States, you may first want to contact your health insurance provider for benefit information and referrals in your area. They can provide you with a list of licensed behavioral health professionals who specialize in treating children and adolescents. Your pediatrician can also refer you to a licensed clinician in your area. You may also ask friends and family for recommendations. The advent of telehealth visits widens your net.

When seeking psychotherapy or mental health care, it is important that the professional you choose have the proper training and licensing. In the US, the professions that are licensed to treat mental health conditions include clinical psychologists, clinical social workers, mental health counselors, clinical nurse practitioners and psychiatrists. Check requirements in your state or country for licensing and professions certified to practice mental health.

Final Thoughts

Our Work Is Not Done

While our children completed their scoliosis treatment years ago, we continue to advocate for you and your children because we understand the importance and power of the unified voice in peer support and advocacy.

Our book showcases the many advances in scoliosis care that have brought a huge impact to the lives of so many girls affected by this condition. However, many challenges remain and we intend to continue our advocacy efforts.

Primary among these challenges is the inequitable access to many of the practices discussed both here and in Curvy Girls' support groups. Scoliosis screening, dissemination of contemporary scoliosis information, and availability of best practices—including peer and family support—remain elusive in too many parts of our country and the world. As a result, far too many children will fail to be diagnosed early in their scoliosis, leaving them to miss out on best treatment practices and endure more prolonged or aggressive measures.

In an effort to bridge that gap, Curvy Girls launched a Diversity, Equity and Inclusion initiative started by Jamiah Bennett. This community of youth leaders examined social dimensions including socioeconomics, gender, religion, race, ethnicity, disability, and geographic accessibility to healthcare. The workgroup also focused specifically on how these elements impact the scoliosis journey and the ability of girls and families to participate in peer support such as Curvy Girls.

We must also continue to advocate for scoliosis-specific exercises, 3D bracing, and low-dose radiation to become standard in the treatment of scoliosis. While physicians and related practitioners are now enthusiastically embracing the benefits of PSSE and 3D bracing, the lack of appropriate health insurance coverage poses a huge challenge. Despite cost-effectiveness in comparison to surgical options, the failure by insurance companies to cover these treatments leaves access dependent upon each family's finances. It is a tragedy that too many children will not have the option to access these treatments.

To address this, professional associations—and families—need to continue to bring forward the national and international research, as well as first-person stories of their impact. Curvy Girls' conferences and social media efforts have included educational forums bringing together professionals and patients to anchor discussions concerning the effectiveness of these treatments. Our advocacy work is bearing fruit. By raising awareness of these valuable treatments, we have helped stimulate interest—and growth in the industry. We are no longer limited to a handful of qualified providers in the US, as we once were.

Finally, we need to do a better job of achieving universal, early screening for scoliosis—whether that occurs in schools, pediatrician offices, and/or through self-screening, such as with the scoliometer or a free phone app such as SpineScreen from Shriners Hospitals for Children. Fewer than half of US states mandate school screenings, so it's important that we promote and ensure evidenced-based screening tools and strategies.

It is our ultimate hope that this book will encourage you to add your voice to our collective efforts by "paying it forward," so others can benefit from your family's experiences: Share something you learned from this book, raise awareness about the importance of early detection and peer support, and ensure that your health providers are familiar with the latest conservative care options so they, too, can become advocates for new standards of care for scoliosis.

We are more together than alone. Let's continue to make a difference together!

In support,

Robin and Terry

Scoliosis Glossary
WORDS EVERY PARENT NEEDS TO KNOW

AIS adolescent idiopathic scoliosis

Apex the maximum point of the scoliosis curve

ApiFix non-fusion surgical system to correct a scoliosis curvature

Asymmetry unevenness between parts of the body as related to scoliosis

Bone Age measurement of physical growth compared to chronological age determined with an X-ray of the left wrist

Boston Brace Original low profile, TLSO-type made of lightweight plastic and specific padding to apply pressure, and relief/cutouts opposite to provide room to correct the spine

Boston Brace 3D low profile, TLSO-type scoliosis brace, made of light weight plastic with specific enhanced built-in pressure areas and opposite relief areas that is custom fabricated from a scan of the patient

Cervical Spine neck vertebrae C1 to C7

Charleston Bending Brace® nighttime "bending brace" made of molded plastic and padding, worn only while sleeping; overcorrects by bending curve in opposite direction

Cobb Angle standard measurement of the spinal curve in scoliosis.

Coronal Plane front or back of the spine sometimes referred to as the frontal plane

Compensatory Curve curve that develops in response to the imbalance produced by the primary curve

Fusion two bones permanently joined

Growth Plate the area near the ends of all long bones in children and adolescents where cartilage slowly changes into bone

Idiopathic Scoliosis spine curvature with no known cause

Kyphosis excessive outward curvature in the upper thoracic spine causing a hunch back

Lordosis inward curvature of the spine causing sway back

Lumbar Spine lower spine vertebrae L1 to L5

Orthotist professional technician who custom makes back braces

Osteoid Osteomia benign bone tumor

PCA Pump device that allows a patient to control the amount of intravenous pain medication received

Physiotherapy Scoliosis Specific Exercises (PSSE) combination of physical therapy methods, such as the BSPTS Rigo Method, Schroth Method, SEAS, that have proven effective in treating scoliosis

Providence Brace low-profile plastic molded brace only worn while sleeping, provides similar correction to daytime braces for mild to moderate curvature

Rigo System Chêneau Brace (RSC)® patented, three-dimensional brace design with open areas that pair with movements associated with scoliosis-specific exercises

Risser Sign grading system for ossification (hardening) of the cartilage of the iliac crest apophysis (growth plate located in the outer edge of the pelvis) which can be helpful to determine skeletal maturity

Sagittal Plane side view of the spine

Sanders Maturity Scale indicator based on left hand X-ray used to determine skeletal maturity

Scoliometer screening tool used to detect trunk asymmetry

Scoliosis musculoskeletal condition that causes lateral curvature of the spine of 10 degrees or more, resulting in a spine that appears S- or C-shaped

Section 504 the part of Americans with Disabilities Act that protects the rights of pre-k through grade 12 students in the education environment

Skeletal Maturity   when bones and spine are finished growing

SpineCor® System   soft TLSO made from cloth and elastic corrective straps used in low to moderate immature curves

Syrinx   cyst within the spinal cord

Thoracic Spine   mid- to upper- spine vertebrae (T1 to T12)

Titanium Rod   metal device used in spinal fusion surgery to correct the curvature of scoliosis

TLSO Brace   lightweight plastic spinal brace that provides key pad placement, putting three-point pressure on the curve to support the thoracic, lumbar, and sacral regions of the spine

Vertebrae   small bones forming the spinal column

Vertebral Body Tethering   fusionless surgical technique that preserves spinal mobility

WCR Brace   three-dimensional brace that maximizes the four Rigo-Chêneau biomechanical principles to correct patient's posture and halt progression of the curve

Acknowledgments

We have a saying in Curvy Girls, "If you've made a difference in one person's life, you've done a great thing." Our journey with helping girls and families affected by scoliosis was enriched by people similarly driven to go the "extra mile." We extend our gratitude to our contributors and advisors who are committed to making a difference.

Jamiah and Cynthia, Alyssa and Jusna, Katelyn and Amy, Mimi and Julie, Intisar and Shahida, Sophie and Cara, and our daughters Leah and Rachel—a heartfelt thank you for allowing us to share your stories in order to help other girls and families know they're not alone.

Curvy Moms Patty Borzner, Sandra Dorton, Regina Papile, Debbie Zenz for sharing your lessons learned.

To our talented and dedicated Mentors Bridget, Emily, Gillian, Jamiah, Jenny, Katelyn, Olivia, and Sara for your undying support while carrying the torch into the next generation.

And we will always be grateful to our Curvy Girls' Mom, Penny Scarangella-Smith. She was more than just a friendly face at monthly meetings. She was a powerful advocate who passionately used her voice to promote low-dose imaging. Penny was among the many heroic front-line nurses, caring for Covid patients daily. Every life lost due to this pandemic is a tragedy; we'd like to take this moment and remember Penny, who lost her life while caring for others.

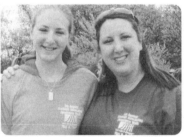

CG Kimberly with her mom, Penny

TO OUR PROFESSIONAL CONTRIBUTORS

James Barci, Craig Eberson, Philip Fischer, A. Noelle Larson, Laurence Mermelstein, Stefano Negrini, Joshua Pahys, Nigel Price, Manuel Rigo, Michael Vitale for generously sharing your medical expertise and support to the Curvy Girls' organization throughout the years.

Mike Mangino, Luke Strikeleather, Grant Wood and James Wynne for your compassion and dedication to improve the quality of scoliosis bracing for our children.

Our sincerest appreciation to Beth Janssen for your vision, passion and dedication to the scoliosis community over the past 18 years. Leading by example, she works tirelessly educating medical communities and supporting Curvy Girls' families. Though she may be small in stature, this remarkable woman is someone we will always look up to. Thank you for your tireless efforts in putting service above self and leaving a lifelong impact on all of our lives.

Gratitude to our Medical Advisor and friend, Marissa Muccio, for the guidance and support you graciously provide to children and families across the globe. We appreciate not only your contribution to this book but your compassionate and astute teachings on scoliosis health.

Ellen Stoltz, wonderful aunt and brilliant teacher, thank you for being a Curvy Girls' guide through the education system.

Aaron Cook and Dana Goldy for sharing your expertise on the value of low-dose radiation and your support to Curvy Girls.

Robyn Rexford, the reason Curvy meetings are soda- and sugar-free, for sharing your common-sense approach to bone health.

Ilene Corina and Robin Moulder for your guidance and work in the field of medical advocacy.

TALENT CONTRIBUTORS

Editor Doug Love for your patience and skill in helping us give voice to our vision.

Tom Emmerson, aka Curvy Dad, of Alternative Graphic Solutions for guiding us in design.

CG Jenna and Mom Patrice Stern for your artistic talents. We are deeply grateful to have had you in our lives early in this journey.

Glenda Torasso, CG Leader of Italy, for bringing to life a vision of scoliosis acceptance and beauty.

Ryan Hershkowitz for your legal expertise and astute advice.

Special acknowledgment to our very own 24/7 personal traveling editor Mike. You're the best!

TO OUR FAMILIES, *who can finally stop asking if the book is done yet!*

Thank you for your patience and allowing us to once again dare greatly to achieve our dreams.

As with everything we've done in our lives, none of this would have been accomplished without the love and technical support from our husbands, Michael and Bobby.

And finally, to all those impacted by scoliosis, we hope that sharing our personal stories has helped you feel less alone. Together, let us continue to make a difference.

Meet the Authors

THERESA E. MULVANEY

The mother of four adult children, Theresa has been an advocate for children with learning disabilities and their families, as well as her current work for those affected by scoliosis. Her youngest daughter's experience with scoliosis led Theresa to becoming a Parent Advocate for Curvy Girls. She devotes countless hours guiding and supporting families around the country. Theresa also works with professionals and medical practices to adopt patient-centered, conservative approaches to scoliosis care.

Theresa and her husband, Bobby, a facilities engineer, reside in Mount Sinai, NY.

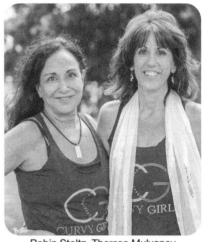

Robin Stoltz, Theresa Mulvaney

ROBIN STOLTZ, LCSW

An educator and Clinical Social Worker for over 35 years, Robin is the mother of two adult children. Her younger child Leah's experience with scoliosis, which inspired her to start Curvy Girls, led Robin to meet with Girls' parents to lend guidance. Robin supports the work of Curvy Girls' mentors overseeing 100+ chapters worldwide. After many years as Deputy Executive Director of a behavioral health center, Robin now has a private practice specializing in adolescents and adults. She holds credentials in addiction disorders and has advanced training in evidence-based approaches to trauma including EMDR and mindfulness.

Robin and her husband, Michael, also a social worker, reside in Smithtown, NY and have traveled the country in their RV joyfully visiting our CG leaders along the way.

Straight Talk Scoliosis – The Journey Continues

To order additional copies of this book and make arrangements for Authors and Curvy Girls speaking engagements:
www.straighttalkscoliosis.com

Also check out:
Finding Curvy Girls
My Scoliosis Journey Coloring and Activity Book

www.curvygirlsscoliosis.com